Eye Care in Developing Nations

Fourth Edition

Larry Schwab, MD

Clinical Professor
Department of Ophthalmology
School of Medicine
West Virginia University
Morgantown, West Virginia, USA

Adjunct Associate Professor
School of Tropical Medicine and Public Health
Tulane University
New Orleans, Louisiana, USA

Research Associate
Dana Center for Preventive Ophthalmology
Wilmer Eye Institute
Johns Hopkins University
Baltimore, Maryland, USA

D0303249

MANSON PUBLISHING

For Martha, who understands, and for Eric, Mark, and Angela, who share the journey.

Love is the greatest healer to be found
Willie Nelson, in his song *Angel Flying Too Close to the Ground*

Photographic credits:

Aravind Hospitals: chapt. 1 facing, 7, 49–54, 56–58, 60, 61, 64, 65, chapt. 6 facing
Harjinder Chana: 108
International Campaign to Ban Landmines: 94
International Centre for Eye Health: chapt. 13 facing, Murray McGavin, 155/Aravind
International Eye Foundation: front cover top insets, chapt. 2 facing, 8–10, 11
Merck Pharmaceuticals: 115
Larry Schwab: front cover, Malawi children, 1–6, 13–22, chapt. 4 facing p, 23–35, chapt. 5 facing, 40–44, 46, 47, 77–80, 80, 83, 84, 86, 89, 92, 93, 95, 96, 100–107, 109–112, chapt. 10 facing, 121, 122, chapt.11 facing, 125–127, 129, 130, 132–134, 144, 146, 147, 149 chapt. 14 half tone, part 3 half tone
Ivan Schwab: 97, 99, 123, 4, 128, 136–143, 145, 150, 153
Martha Schwab (original drawings, color enhanced and modified by Kate Nardoni): 12, 22, 38, 55, 59, 62, 63, 68, 70, 72, 74–76, 81, 83, 85, 87, 98, 151, 152, 154, 157–169, 172
Marty Spencer: 48, 148
Jim Standefer: cover, lower right inset, 36, 66, 67, 69, 71, 170, 171
Jeff Watson: 117, 119
World Health Organization: 81, 82, 88, 90, 91, 113, 114, 118, 120, 131

Copyright © 2007 Manson Publishing Ltd

UK edition: ISBN 978-1-84076-084-2
Indian sub-continent edition: ISBN 978-1-84076-103-0

A CIP catalogue record for this book is available from the British Library.

For full details of all Manson Publishing titles please write to:
Manson Publishing Ltd, 73 Corringham Road, London NW11 7DL, UK.
Tel: +44(0)20 8905 5150
Fax: +44(0)20 8201 9233
Website: www.mansonpublishing.com

Commissioning editor: Jill Northcott
Project manager and book design: Ayala Kingsley
Copy editor: Alan Bellinger
Illustration: Cactus Design and Illustration
Colour reproduction: Tenon & Polert Colour Scanning Ltd, Hong Kong
Printed by: New Era Printing Co Ltd, Hong Kong

Contents

Contents

PART 2

Blinding disorders and eye care

PART 3

Ophthalmology backgrounder

PART 4

Appendices

Foreword

The prevention of blindness is known to be one of the most cost-effective health interventions that can be undertaken. It should start at the individual, family, and community levels. Primary eye care, as part of primary health care, has thus been strongly advocated by the World Health Organization's Program for the Prevention of Blindness and Deafness in its long-standing partnership with the International Eye Foundation and other non-governmental organizations. To be meaningful, primary eye care must respond to local needs and resources and must use opportunities for community support. This implies priority for basic eye care, often in a difficult setting of resource constraints in developing countries.

This book responds particularly well to the need for practical, innovative, and affordable solutions to bring eye care to those populations most in need in the developing world. The most common ocular disorders and their management are described, including public health perspectives and appropriate guidelines.

It is a pleasure and encouragement to note the continuing great success and demand for the practical guidance to eye care given in this book. The time has now come to provide the fourth edition, which includes a number of useful updates.

The book contributes greatly to increasing the access to basic eye care services in developing countries. Such services, along with appropriate public health interventions, constitute the key to eliminating unnecessary visual loss in future generations. The existence of effective public/private partnerships for the prevention of blinding diseases, along with the rapid progress of 'Vision 2020: the Right to Sight' global movement should make it possible to achieve that goal.

Bjorn Thylefors M.D., Ph.D., FRCOpht
Director, Mectizan Donation Program, Decatur, Georgia

About this book

The text of this book has been written for mid-level eye health care workers. For some people who will use it in the classroom and as a reference, this book may be elementary; for others, it may be too complex. The aim is to present the major causes of blindness and visual impairment in a concise and accessible format. Ophthalmologists have found it to be useful as a resource guide.

Eye Care in Developing Nations is divided into three sections: Part 1, *Public health ophthalmology*; Part 2, *Blinding disorders and eye care*; and Part 3, *Ophthalmology Backgrounder*. Part 1 introduces concepts in public health ophthalmology, an area that deserves more emphasis in the realm of blindness prevention. Part 3, a basic primer in anatomy, physiology, and the ocular examination, is primarily intended for non-physician eye-care workers in developing nations. People who seek more complete information on ocular anatomy and physiology should consult a standard ophthalmology textbook.

Ophthalmologists will likely find Part 2, the clinically oriented section, the most useful in their practical efforts to prevent blindness and restore sight, especially for those who are unfamiliar with 'tropical' ophthalmic conditions.

The glossary, which for easy reference now comes before the first chapter, has been expanded from the third edition, as have the appendices. Key resource organizations, both local and international, are described in Appendix G, and an address list of these and others is listed in Appendix H.

Clinical points of special importance appear in boldface italics. Measurements are listed in metric units. American units may be given for convenience in parentheses subsequently; for example, a normal visual acuity would be given as 6/6 (20/20), that is, meters first, feet second.

Algorithms and treatment schedules follow World Health Organization guidelines. Vision 2020 recommendations are included in the text. International Agency for the Prevention of Blindness and International Council of Ophthalmology information is also included in the International Agencies appendix.

Suggestions on how to improve future editions of this title would be appreciated. You may reach the author through www.iefusa.org.

Preface

People do not go blind by the millions.
They go blind one by one, each in an individual and tragic way.
Sir John Wilson

'tis the gift to be simple
'tis the gift to be free
'tis the gift to come down where we ought to be
Shaker tune *Simple Gifts*, Joseph Brackett, Jr.

Millions of blind people live in our world. They do not go blind by the millions, as the visionary Sir John Wilson, blind himself, once said. If you have ever known a blind person, then you are likely aware of the enormous physical, social, psychological, and economic toll that blindness inflicts. But millions? Is it really possible to comprehend the magnitude of this silent catastrophe?

The numbers are staggering: 37 million people blind and another 124 million with low vision. A total of 161 million are visually impaired. One person goes blind every five seconds, on average, and one child goes blind every minute.

At least 75% of all blindness is either reversible, in the case of cataract, or preventable, as with trachoma and external eye infections, for example. Ninety percent of all new blindness occurs in the developing world. Most of those people are impoverished and have limited access to eye care. Most are adults, but millions are children. Who among us can condone the tragedy of childhood blindness that could have been prevented?

Should the international health care community, public health specialists, administrators, political leaders, and concerned citizens forge a social contract with those who are blind and people who are at high risk of blindness? I believe they should. Many of us already have, as evidenced by the non-governmental organizations and international agencies described in the resource appendices of this edition. I believe it is an ethical and moral imperative that everything that can be done to prevent blindness and restore sight should be done.

The intent of this book is simple and clear. *Eye Care in Developing Nations* was first published in 1987 for medical assistants, clinical officers, and nurses training and working in eye care in Africa. Two subsequent English editions followed in 1990 and 1999. The title has been translated into Chinese, French, Tibetan, and Vietnamese editions.

This fourth edition has been expanded and updated. New text, treatment algorithms, and diagnostic criteria have been added. This is the first edition in which color plates have been published. The varied photographs in this edition depict both common and rare ocular conditions. Suggestions of colleagues and co-workers have been taken into consideration in revising and expanding the text and illustrations.

Somewhere today on the Gangetic Plain of northern India and southern Nepal, a child, blind from corneal scarring secondary to vitamin A deficiency and measles, will perish from starvation. A teenager in Indochina will detonate a landmine with her innocent footfall while walking to school, taking her legs and her eyesight. An African elder, his hair white with the dignity of age and his pupils white with mature cataracts, will die, his sight-restoring surgery never performed because he did not have access to eye care. An indigenous Latin American, severely sub-sighted, will forego a trip to the eye specialist for treatment of her glaucoma for lack of bus fare as she is slowly blinded by her disease.

There is simultaneous tragedy and hope in these human snapshots. There is tragedy because preventable blindness persists in a bountiful world, one of unequal resource distribution. Hope, because in each instance, blindness could have been prevented.

It is in the spirit of hope that this book can assist the international efforts and local action in preventing blindness and restoring sight in disadvantaged populations.

Larry Schwab

Acknowledgments

The author and publisher gratefully acknowledge the generous assistance, friendly advice, and constructive criticism of these colleagues, friends, organizations, and family:

Sue Stevens of the International Centre for Eye Health was wonderfully supportive and encouraging in the preparation of this edition. Her gift of time and energy was enormously helpful.

Ayala Kingsley of Manson Publishing Ltd, was unstinting with her professional talent and hard work. Her sense of purpose and good humor also contributed marvelously.

Aravind Hospitals, India, for collaboration and assistance in Chapter 2
John Barrows, International Eye Foundation (IEF), for co-authoring Chapter 2
Paul Courtright, KCCO, Tanzania, for suggestions and critique of Chapter 10
Jill Dorman, for indexing
John Forder, Manson Publishing, for proof-reading the final draft
Ken Gustavsen, Merck Pharmaceuticals, for generous support to make possible the distribution of this title to eye health workers serving underserved people.
Tom Jackson, Manson Publishing, for final revisions and review
Susan Lewallen, KCCO, Tanzania, for suggestions and encouragement
Michael Manson, Manson Publishing, for his enthusiastic support of this title, blindness prevention, and sight restoration
Kate Nardoni, for color artwork
Ramachandra Pararagasegaram, WHO, for suggestions and IAPB/WHO data
Raheem Rahmathullah, IEF, for co-authoring Chapter 2
Serge Resnikoff, WHO, for suggestions and WHO data
Martha Schwab, for the original line drawings
Victoria Sheffield, IEF, for co-authoring Chapter 2
Marty Spencer, Seva Foundation, for suggestions on Chapter 5
Jim Standefer, for valuable critique of Chapter 6
Bjorn Thylefors, Mectizan Donation Program, for critical review of Chapter 9 and Foreword
Jack Whitcher, Proctor Foundation, for critical reading and suggestions on Chapter 7

Credits:
Blindness and low vision data: World Health Organization, 2002

Cardiff University Information Services

Law Library

Request No: CP010784   Due Date: ~~0711112~~ 06/12/12.

Item Details: Eye care in developing nations / Schwab

If recalled before the above date, it must be returned immediately.

Failure to return the item promptly will result in an automatic additional charge for renewal.

This item must not be lent to another person.   Responsibility for the return rests with the signatory of the loan.

This item must be returned to the Law Library before leaving Cardiff for vacations.

PATEL, J.   (ILL) due back 7/11/12

Glossary

We shall not cease from exploration
And the end of all our exploring
Will be to arrive where we started
And to know the place for the first time.
T.S. Eliot, *Four Quartets*

It is a simple matter to make things complicated;
it is much more complicated to make matters simple.
Meyer's Law

A

absolute glaucoma End-stage glaucoma. A condition in which there is no light perception (NLP) and usually pain, often severe, from a glaucomatous process.

accommodation A change in the power of the crystalline lens that allows the eye to focus at near. Accommodation is accomplished by contraction of the ciliary muscle with relaxation of the ciliary zonules and thickening of the lens. The eye's ability to accommodate decreases naturally with age.

AC IOL Anterior chamber intraocular lens.

acuity Visual acuity.

acute In medical use, sudden or immediate.

adenopathy Enlargement of lymph node(s); also called lymphadenopathy.

adnexa Ocular eyelids, lacrimal system, extraocular muscles, orbit, and other surrounding structures of the eyeball.

afferent pupillary defect The 'swinging flashlight' sign; a test with a focal light to determine if posterior segment or optic nerve disease is present. In the affected eye, the pupil may be sluggish to constrict to light and will not constrict further and may even dilate when the stimulus of light in the fellow eye is removed and 'swung' to the affected eye; an important clinical test.

agonist A drug that stimulates physiological activity.

AIDS Autoimmune Deficiency Syndrome: a disease complex caused by a specific retrovirus (HIV) that attacks the immune system, resulting in opportunistic infections (including Herpes zoster and Kaposi's sarcoma).

akinesia Paralysis of movement of the eye or eyelids by paralyzing the extraocular or orbicularis muscles using local anesthetic.

allopathy A system of health care practice that attempts to produce a condition opposite to the disease state in an attempt to cure the disease. Compare homeopathy.

amblyopia Failure of vision to develop properly, frequently due to strabismus or anisometropia; sometimes called 'lazy eye.'

AMD Age-related macular degeneration. See macular degeneration.

ametropia A refractive error.

anesthesia Loss of sensation, especially absence of pain, after administering an anesthetic drug. Injury to sensory nerves may also produce anesthesia.

angle Junction of the iris and the cornea in the anterior chamber.

aniseikonia A difference in the size of ocular image between the two eyes, caused by aphakia in one eye only.

anisometropia A condition where there are two or more diopters of difference in the refractive error between the two eyes.

antagonist A drug that neutralizes the action of another substance.

anterior chamber (AC) Space between the cornea and the iris that is filled with aqueous fluid.

anterior segment The front part of the eye, including the cornea, surgical limbus, anterior chamber, iris, and lens with its attachments (zonules).

anterior uveitis Inflammation (uveitis) of the iris (iritis) or ciliary body (cyclitis), or both (iridocyclitis).

antimetabolite Any of various drugs used in chemotherapy of cancer; in glaucoma filtering surgery, one of several drugs that may be used to intentionally delay healing and closure of the surgical fistula that is being used to drain aqueous fluid and thus to lower intraocular pressure.

antipersonnel landmine (APL) In-ground explosive weapon, triggered by pressure or vibration. Used to deny access to large areas, they are usually left in place after deployment, where they kill, maim, or blind thousands of civilians annually.

aphake A person with unilateral or bilateral aphakia.

aphakia The condition of the eye without a lens, usually as a result of cataract extraction.

aphakic spectacles Highly convex (plus) lenses.

APL Antipersonnel landmine.

applanation A form of tonometry in which the force required to flatten a small area of the central cornea is measured.

aqueous (aqueous fluid; aqueous humor) The consistency of water that fills the anterior chamber, produced by the epithelium of the ciliary body.

argon laser Laser instrument used to treat diabetic retinopathy (pan retinal photocoagulation), primary open-angle glaucoma (trabeculoplasty), acute angle-closure glaucoma (iridotomy), and other intraocular disease states.

Arlt's line Characteristic tarsal eyelid scar in trachoma.

asymptomatic Without symptoms.

asthenopia Mild ocular discomfort often due to refractive error in healthy eyes; commonly called 'eye strain.'

astigmatism (Greek, 'without a point') Refractive error due to a non-spherical corneal surface.

autoclave A metal chamber equipped to use steam or gas under high pressure and temperature to sterilize surgical instruments.

B

background diabetic retinopathy (BDR)
Changes in the retinal vascular system that can occur in diabetes mellitus including microaneurysms and intraretinal hemorrhages.

BDR Background diabetic retinopathy.

bifocal A compound spectacle lens divided horizontally, with the lower part for near vision and the upper part for distance vision.

bilateral Both right and left sides (e.g., right and left eyes).

binocular With both eyes together.

biomicroscope See slit lamp.

Bitot's spot A characteristic white spot on the temporal conjunctiva in chronic vitamin A deficiency.

bleb Skin or tissue elevated by fluid or air. In ophthalmology, the usual context is a conjunctival bleb into which aqueous is drained after successful glaucoma surgery.

blepharitis Infection or inflammation of the eyelids, often due to the bacterium *Staphylococcus aureus*.

blindness The World Health Organization's definition of blindness is a visual acuity of less than 3/60 (20/400), or counting fingers at 3 m, in the better eye.

blindness prevention A broad category of eye health-care activities including ophthalmic medical and surgical therapy, control of infectious ocular disease, improved nutrition to cure, prevent, or forestall blindness, and public health education.

blindness prevention committee
A group of experts in health care, including health planners, administrators, ophthalmic auxiliaries, and ophthalmologists, that coordinates and plans national blindness prevention activities.

bulbar Pertaining to the eyeball.

buphthalmos (Greek, 'ox eye') Enlarged eye resulting from congenital glaucoma.

C

canaliculitis Infection of the lacrimal canaliculi.

canaliculus (plural: canaliculi) A tiny tubular structure that drains tears from the lacrimal puncti (on both upper and lower eyelids) to the lacrimal sac.

canthus (plural: canthi) The junction of the upper and lower eyelids. The nasal junction is called the medial canthus and the temporal junction is called the lateral canthus.

capsule Lens capsule.

cardinal positions of gaze The six points to which a patient's gaze are directed to test extraocular muscle function. The positions are right and up, right, right and down, left and up, left, and left and down.

caruncle A small fleshy elevation of conjunctival tissue in the medial canthus.

cataract A density or opacity of the lens, usually causing visual disability or blindness. Cataract is the major cause of blindness worldwide.

cautery Application of a heated probe to bleeding vessels to stop the bleeding.

cc Cubic centimeter; 1 cc is equivalent in volume to 1 milliliter.

cells and flare Signs seen in the anterior chamber with the slit lamp usually indicating anterior uveitis (iritis).

CF Counts fingers; a measure of visual acuity.

chalazion Small firm chronic eyelid mass that results from a blocked eyelid gland.

chemosis Edema and swelling of the conjunctiva and Tenon's capsule.

Chlamydia Microorganism (a bacterium) that causes trachoma.

chorioretinitis Inflammation (uveitis) of the choroid and retina.

choroid Vascular layer of uveal tissue located between the retina and sclera.

choroiditis Inflammation (uveitis) of the choroid.

chronic In medical use, long term or relatively unresolvable.

cicatricial Referring to the scarring process.

cicatrix Scar.

ciliary body The ring of uveal tissue and muscle posterior to the iris.

ciliary flush Blood vessel injection in the sclera at the limbus.

clinical officer Auxiliary health care worker trained in the practice of general medicine. With training in ophthalmology, the CO becomes an ophthalmic clinical officer.

cm Centimeter; 1/100th of a meter.

CME Cystoid macular edema.

CO Clinical officer.

community health worker A primary health care worker who lives and works in a village or community.

complicated cataract Lens opacity associated with or caused by ocular disease or injury.

complication An unexpected and unwanted occurrence during or resulting from surgery or therapy.

cone A type of photoreceptor cell in the retina that detects colored light and functions most efficiently in high illumination (bright light). The cones serve light and color vision and visual acuity. Compare *rod*.

confrontation field test A simple method of measuring peripheral vision and the visual field.

congenital Referring to conditions or diseases present at birth.

conjunctiva Transparent tissue covering the sclera and inner surfaces of the eyelids.

conjunctivitis Inflammation or infection of the conjunctiva.

contraindication A sign or symptom suggesting that a particular therapy should be avoided or discontinued. For example, topical corticosteroids are contraindicated in the presence of dendritic corneal ulcer due to herpes simplex.

contusion Blunt non-penetrating injury. Contusion to the eye may result in serious extraocular and intraocular injury.

cornea Transparent tissue at the front of the eye.

corneal abrasion A scratch of the corneal epithelium.

corneal endothelium The layer of cells that covers the inner surface of the cornea and helps to maintain proper fluid balance within the cornea.

corneal epithelium The outermost layer of the cornea that provides protection against infection and injury and a smooth refracting surface for the eye.

corneal laceration A tearing or slicing wound penetrating into the cornea or through the cornea into the anterior chamber.

corneal ulcer Localized infection of the cornea, which may cause permanent corneal scarring and blindness.

cortex Lens tissue surrounding the nucleus and covered by the lens capsule.

cortico- Prefix indicating lens cortex involvement, e.g., corticonuclear.

corticosteroids A group of hormones occurring naturally in the human body that have important therapeutic value in treating inflammation. The term is frequently shortened to 'steroids.'

couching Traditional ophthalmic surgical practice in which the cataract is dislocated into the vitreous cavity by an instrument inserted in the eye or by digital or instrument pressure to the ocular surface. Couching is dangerous and often followed by serious intraocular complications. It is not in standard or widespread use in developing nations.

cryoextraction Removal of a cataract with an instrument that freezes and adheres to the lens.

cryoextractor Portable instrument for performing cryoextraction.

crystalline lens Natural, transparent structure behind the iris that focuses light onto the retina.

curettage Removal of tissue by scraping with a sharp instrument.

cyclitis Inflammation (uveitis) of the ciliary body.

cyclodialysis Surgical or traumatic separation of the ciliary body and choroid from the sclera.

cycloplegic Drug that dilates the pupil and temporarily paralyzes the ciliary body.

cystoid macular edema (CME) Fluid in the macula and fovea that results in decreased and distorted central vision; CME may follow cataract surgery, other intraocular surgery, and trauma.

cystotome A narrow metal instrument with a hooked, pointed tip used for opening the lens capsule.

D

dacryo- Prefix referring to the lacrimal system.

dacryocystitis Infection of the lacrimal sac.

debride To remove diseased or injured tissue or foreign material, usually by sharp dissection.

dendrite Characteristic branching pattern of herpes simplex corneal ulcer.

diabetes mellitus (DM) Systemic abnormality of sugar and carbohydrate metabolism. Diabetes may affect retinal vessels and cause retinopathy.

differential diagnosis List of possible underlying causes (diagnoses) of a particular clinical condition.

diopter A unit of measurement of optical power. A 1 diopter lens brings light to a point focus at a distance of 1 meter.

direct ophthalmoscope A hand-held instrument that provides an upright, monocular view of the ocular fundus.

disc Optic disc.

disc cupping Normal central depression in the optic disc (physiological cupping). Deep cupping with optic atrophy is usually due to glaucoma (glaucomatous cupping).

discission Surgical opening of the lens capsule (anterior or posterior).

DM Diabetes mellitus.

dresser A medical auxiliary. When trained in ophthalmology, the dresser is an ophthalmic dresser.

dry AMD Atrophic age-related macular degeneration.

dysfunction Impaired functioning of an organ.

E

ECCE Extracapsular cataract extraction.

ecchymosis Blood under the skin causing it to appear dark and swollen; a 'bruise.'

ectropion The condition of an eyelid turned outward from the globe.

edema Abnormal fluid resulting from injury or disease that causes tissue swelling.

e.g. (Latin, 'exempli gratia') For example.

EKC Epidemic keratoconjunctivitis.

emmetropia The refractive state of an eye that is able to focus correctly; opposite of ametropia.

endemic Usually present in a population at all times.

endophthalmitis Internal infection or inflammation of the eyeball. Endophthalmitis is a very serious condition, often resulting in loss of sight and sometimes requiring enucleation.

endothelium Innermost tissue lining.

end-stage glaucoma (see absolute glaucoma) A condition of high pressure, no light perception, and usually pain, sometimes severe, from a glaucomatous process.

entropion An eyelid that is turned inward toward the globe; common in trachoma. The eyelashes may also touch the cornea (trichiasis).

enucleation Surgical removal of the eyeball.

epidemic Occurring and spreading rapidly, usually by infection, in a large number of people at the same time.

epidemic keratoconjunctivitis (EKC) A contagious viral conjunctivitis, usually bilateral, affecting both the corneae and conjunctivae.

epidemiology Science and study of the distribution of diseases.

epilation Removal of eyelashes by pulling out with forceps or tweezers.

epithelium A covering or top layer of tissue.

erysiphake Small, simple surgical instrument used in intracapsular cataract extraction. The erysiphake is attached to the cataract by suction, and the cataract is removed from the eye manually.

esotropia Misalignment of the eyes with one eye turned inward.

etiology The cause or origin of a medical problem.

eversion Turning outward. The upper eyelid is everted in various procedures to expose the conjunctiva and tarsus.

evisceration The surgical removal of intraocular contents leaving the scleral shell; compare with enucleation.

exotropia Misalignment of the eyes with one eye turned outward.

extracapsular cataract extraction (ECCE) Surgical removal of the contents of the cataractous lens, except the posterior capsule, which is left in place.

extraocular Outside the eyeball. Usually refers to tissues within and surrounding the orbit.

F

farsightedness Hyperopia.

fistula A passage or opening in body tissue.

fixate To gaze steadily at a visual target.

flare Light beam of the slit lamp visible in the anterior chamber, indicating presence of protein. A sign of inflammation (anterior uveitis).

fluorescein Yellow-green dye used in diagnosing ocular surface injuries and diseases.

focal grid Application of regular argon laser burns to the central retina in diabetic retinopathy to reduce swelling and fluid in the retina, thereby improving visual acuity.

follicles Small, whitish, isolated elevations of the conjunctiva, especially tarsal conjunctiva, seen in trachoma, ocular viral infections, and drug reactions.

fornix (plural: fornices) The potential space lined by conjunctival tissue where the eyelid conjunctiva and bulbar conjunctiva meet beneath the upper and lower eyelids.

fovea Tiny depression in the center of the macula; contains the highest density of cone photoreceptors in the retina.

functional vision In a visually disabled person, visual acuity and/or peripheral vision sufficient for the person to carry out normal activities.

fundus Back surface of the interior of the eye.

fungus (plural: fungi) An organism that usually gains its nutrients by absorbing dead organic matter. A few fungi are parasites and feed on living hosts; some of these can cause serious ocular complications.

G

GET 2020 Abbreviation for name of Global Elimination of Trachoma by the Year 2020.

glare Overly bright light or light reflection, which can interfere with vision.

glaucoma Intraocular disease characterized by intraocular pressure sufficiently high to cause damage to the optic nerve and retina. Glaucoma often results in blindness and is a leading cause of blindness and low vision worldwide.

globe The eyeball without its surrounding structures.

GNID Gram-negative intracellular Diplococcus. *Neisseria gonorrhoeae* is a GNID.

gonioscopy A method of examining the angle and trabecular meshwork with a special lens (goniolens) placed on the anesthetized corneal surface.

goniotomy An operation performed for congenital glaucoma in which the trabecular meshwork is incised.

Graefe knife A precision surgical knife with a long sharp blade used for creating incisions across the anterior chamber of the eye between the cornea and sclera prior to cataract extraction.

Gram's stain Laboratory chemical process of dye staining to identify bacteria.

granuloma Elevated, non-infectious mass in conjunctiva, skin, or internal organs that results from chronic inflammation.

granulomatous Referring to disease processes that produce granulomas (e.g., tuberculosis).

H

Hansen's disease Another term for leprosy; named after Gerhard Armauer Hansen, who identified the disease-causing bacterium.

haptic The arm of an intraocular lens, used to grasp it and position it securely in the eye.

harmful eye practices Ocular treatment by traditional healers or non-medical individuals with plant or animal products, thermal cautery, or mechanical means, causing temporary or permanent damage to the eye.

hemostasis Control of bleeding.

herbalist Traditional healer who uses plant products to cure, treat, or manage disease (including ocular disease) or mental illness.

Herbert's pits Small depressions resulting from trachoma scarring that are found at the superior limbus.

herpes simplex virus (HSV) A virus capable of infecting skin, conjunctiva, and corneal epithelium; may cause permanent corneal scarring.

Hg Mercury. Tonometry measures intra-ocular pressure as the weight of a column of mercury in millimeters.

HIV Human Immunodeficiency Virus: a retrovirus that attacks the immune system, resulting in AIDS.

homeopathy A system of therapeutics in which diseases are treated by small doses of drugs capable of producing in healthy persons symptoms such as those of the disease to be treated.

hordeolum (stye) Acute infection at the eyelid margin, frequently caused by *Staphylococcus*.

HSV Herpes simplex virus.

hypermature cataract A very advanced cataract with a swollen, milky appearance.

hyperopia Refractive error corrected with plus (convex) lens. Visual acuity is good at distance but poor at near; also known as farsightedness.

hypertropia Turning upward of one eye when the other is looking straight ahead.

hyphema Blood in the anterior chamber of the eye. Hyphema may be caused by trauma or may follow intraocular surgery and some intraocular diseases.

hypopyon White blood cells (pus) in the anterior chamber of the eye caused by inflammation or infection.

hypotony Low intraocular pressure.

HZO Herpes zoster ophthalmicus. Infection of the first division of the fifth cranial nerve (CN V) with herpes zoster virus.

I

I and C Incision and curettage.

I and D Incision and drainage.

ICCE Intracapsular cataract extraction.

i.e. (Latin, 'id est') In other words.

incidence The number of new cases of a disease as a proportion of the number of persons at risk over a specified period of time.

indentation A type of tonometry in which the amount of corneal indentation produced by a fixed weight is measured.

inflammatory membrane Layer of tissue secondary to inflammation that can form on the conjunctiva in severe viral conjunctival infection.

injection In blood vessels of the eye, the state of being congested or swollen.

intracapsular cataract extraction (ICCE) Removal of the cataract within and including its capsule.

intraocular Within the eyeball.

intraocular lens (IOL) A permanent plastic optical lens placed in the eye following cataract surgery.

intraocular pressure (IOP) The natural firmness of the eyeball that results from the dynamic secretion and resorption of aqueous fluid.

IOFB Intraocular foreign body.

IOL Intraocular lens.

IOP Intraocular pressure.

iridectomy Surgical removal of a small piece of iris during intraocular surgery to produce an opening from the anterior chamber to the posterior chamber.

iridocyclitis Inflammation (uveitis) of the iris and ciliary body.

iridoplegia Paralysis of the pupil.

iridotomy A small surgical hole created in the iris; may be performed with a laser instrument.

iris Flat ring of uveal tissue in front of the lens.

iris bombé Bowing forward of the mid-iris when the pupil is adhered to the anterior lens capsule; associated with secondary glaucoma.

iris prolapse Iris tissue that protrudes from an opening in the eye; may result from trauma, infection, or intraocular surgery.

iritis Inflammation of the iris (uveitis).

IU International unit.

K

keratic precipitates Tiny deposits on the corneal endothelium, sometimes seen in severe anterior uveitis.

keratitis Inflammation or infection of the cornea.

keratoconjunctivitis Inflammation or infection of the cornea and conjunctiva.

keratomalacia Softening and melting of the cornea, frequently associated with vitamin A deficiency, other micronutrient deficiencies, protein-energy malnutrition, and starvation.

KP Keratic precipitate.

kwashiorkor Protein starvation. Kwashiorkor occurring together with marasmus is referred to as protein-energy malnutrition.

L

lacrimal Referring to the tear system.

lacrimal gland Small gland of the superior temporal anterior orbit that produces tears.

lacrimal sac Cavity of the lacrimal drainage system that collects tears.

lagophthalmos Failure of the eyelids to close normally and completely.

laser Abbreviation for Light Amplification by Stimulated Emission of Radiation; instrument using light energy for ocular surgery.

lavage Irrigation.

LE Left eye.

lens In the eye, the encapsulated transparent ocular tissue (crystalline lens) suspended by the zonules behind the iris and pupil that focuses light on the retina. When used as the term intraocular lens (IOL), refers to an artificial plastic replacement for the natural lens.

lens capsule Envelope covering the crystalline lens of the eye and fusing with the ciliary zonules.

lensometer Optical instrument used to determine the optical strength of lenses and eyeglasses.

leproma (plural: lepromata) Nodule in skin or on the eye resulting from leprosy infection.

lepromatous Pertaining to leprosy.

leprosy A chronic, slowly progressive, infectious disease caused by *Mycobacterium leprae*.

lesion Pathological or traumatic change in tissue or organ that may result in impairment of function.

leukoma White opaque scar in the cornea.

levator muscle Upper eyelid muscle, primarily responsible for elevation of the eyelid.

light perception Visual acuity term meaning the ability of the eye to see only light.

light projection Visual acuity term meaning the ability of the patient to point to the source and direction of light directed into the pupil.

limbal Of the limbus.

limbus The junction between cornea and sclera. The superior limbus, where the eye is most often opened for intraocular surgery, is sometimes referred to as the surgical limbus.

loupe Magnifying glass or spectacles that aid in ocular examination and in performing surgery.

low vision A classification of visual acuity; less than 6/18 (20/60) but equal to or better than 3/60 (20/400).

lues Syphilis.

luxation Dislocation of the crystalline lens.

LVD Low-vision device.

lymphadenopathy Enlargement of lymph node(s).

lysis Dissolution or breaking up.

M

m Meter

macula (plural: maculae) Small central anatomic area of the retina that provides detailed central vision; also, a spot scar of the anterior cornea.

macular Referring to the retinal macula.

macular degeneration Deterioration or breaking down of the macula, usually accompanied by decreased visual acuity; most commonly due to aging.

marasmus Calorie starvation. Marasmus occurring together with kwashiorkor is referred to as protein-energy malnutrition.

MDT Multidrug therapy.

measles Acute viral infectious disease affecting mucous membranes, conjunctiva, cornea, respiratory system, and gastrointestinal tract; responsible for high infant mortality and childhood blindness in populations with protein-energy malnutrition and vitamin A deficiency.

media A collective term for the cornea, aqueous, lens, and vitreous.

medical assistant Auxiliary health care worker trained in the practice of general medicine. When trained in ophthalmology, the medical assistant is an ophthalmic medical assistant.

melanoma Malignant pigmented tumor that can occur in ocular tissue.

mg Milligram; 1/1000th of a gram.

microfilariae *Onchocerca volvulus* larvae; cause of onchocerciasis.

micropannus Very small network of vessels on cornea of ocular surface sometimes seen in inflammatory or infectious conditions, e.g., trachoma.

minus lens Concave lens.

miosis Constriction of the pupil.

miotic Drug that causes miosis.

mitomycin C An antimetabolite that can be used in filtering surgery for glaucoma to intentionally prevent or delay closure that would normally occur upon healing of the fistula.

ml Milliliter; 1/1000th of a liter. Equivalent in volume to 1 cubic centimeter.

mm Millimeter; 1/10th of a centimeter; 1/1000th of a meter.

mobile eye unit Team consisting of vehicle, equipment, supplies, ophthalmic medical auxiliary, assistant, and driver, that provides ophthalmic services, including surgery, to people living in underserved areas; often based at a district or regional hospital.

monocular One eye only.

Morgagnian cataract Hypermature cataract in which the nucleus is floating in degenerated liquefied cortex.

-morphic Suffix meaning shape or form.

mydriasis Dilation of the pupil.

mydriatic Drug that causes mydriasis.

myopia Refractive error corrected by minus (concave) lenses. Visual acuity is good at near but poor at distance; also known as nearsightedness.

N

NaCl Sodium chloride (salt).

nasally In ophthalmology, in the medial direction; toward the nose.

nasolacrimal duct Small channel through which tears drain from the lacrimal sac into the nose.

Nd:YAG laser A type of laser instrument (named for its neodymium, yttrium, aluminum, and garnet light source). A primary use is to create an opening in a clouded posterior capsule after extracapsular cataract surgery with posterior chamber intraocular lens implantation.

nearsightedness Myopia.

nebula (plural: nebulae) A mild scar of the anterior cornea.

neovascularization Growth or proliferation of abnormal new blood vessels.

nevus Darkly pigmented spot that can occur on skin or mucous membranes, including conjunctiva.

night blindness Inability to see properly in dim illumination; often a symptom of vitamin A deficiency in children.

NLP No Light Perception.

nucleus Firm tissue in the central core of the lens.

NV Near vision.

nyctalopia Night blindness.

nystagmus An involuntary, rapid, rhythmic movement of the eyeball.

O

occlude To block or cover.

occlusion Act of blocking or covering.

ocular Referring to the eye.

ocular media A collective term for the cornea, aqueous, lens, and vitreous. Also referred to simply as the media.

ocular surface External aspect of the eyeball, including cornea and conjunctiva.

oculist Alternative term for ophthalmologist in Britain and in some former British colonies.

OD (Latin, 'oculus dexter') Right eye.

onchocerciasis (river blindness) Blinding microfilarial disease caused by *Onchocerca volvulus* and transmitted by *Simulium* black flies, affecting skin, internal organs, and eyes.

ophthalmia neonatorum Ocular infection in newborns frequently caused by *Neisseria gonorrhoeae* (gonococcal keratoconjunctivitis) or *Chlamydia trachomatis*.

ophthalmic Pertaining to the eye.

ophthalmic clinical officer An auxiliary health worker trained in ophthalmology; in some countries may be called ophthalmic medical assistant.

ophthalmologist Physician (medical doctor) trained to perform medical and surgical treatment of the eyes.

ophthalmology Science and study of medical and surgical therapy of the eye.

ophthalmoscope Instrument for examination of the eye and ocular fundus.

optic disc Optic nerve as seen by ophthalmoscopy at its attachment to the posterior eyeball.

optician Person who manufactures, fits, and repairs optical aids, including eyeglasses and contact lenses.

optics Science and study of lenses, light, and effects on vision.

optometrist Non-physician professional trained in refraction, optics, and fitting of optical aids.

optotype Figure, number, letter, or character on the standard visual acuity chart.

orbicularis muscle Oval sphincter muscle surrounding the eyelids; a supporting muscle for the ocular adnexa.

orbit Bony cavity that protects the globe and supporting structures.

OS (Latin, 'oculus sinister') Left eye.

P

pandemic Epidemic occurring over a wide geographic area.

pan retinal photocoagulation (PRP) Treatment with a laser instrument, usually the argon laser, of the mid- and far periphery of the retina with microscopic burns, usually for diabetic retinopathy.

palpebral Pertaining to an eyelid.

pannus Abnormal vascular network on conjunctiva or cornea; results from infection or injury.

papilla (plural: papillae) Tiny tufts of blood vessels appearing diffusely red in conjunctiva. They occur in ocular surface infection and trauma.

paracentesis Removal of fluid from the anterior chamber for therapy or to establish a diagnosis by culturing for microorganisms.

PAS Peripheral anterior synechiae.

pathologic Abnormality present; not normal.

pellagra Nutritional deficiency syndrome secondary to micronutrient deficiency niacin and characterized by the three Ds: dermatitis; diarrhea, and dementia,

PBL Prevention of blindness.

PC Posterior chamber.

PC IOL Posterior chamber intraocular lens.

PCO Posterior capsular opacity; refers to clouding or opacity of the posterior capsule (which supports the implanted posterior chamber intraocular lens) following extracapsular cataract extraction.

PEM Protein-energy malnutrition.

perforation Hole. In ophthalmology, perforation refers to a hole through cornea or sclera into the intraocular space as a result of injury, infection, or disease.

perimetry Formal testing and mapping of the visual field.

peripheral anterior synechiae A condition in which the iris adheres to the cornea at or near the angle in the periphery of the anterior chamber.

pH A scale expressing the acidic or basic nature of a substance. A pH of 7.0 is neutral; below pH 7.0 is increasingly acidic; above pH 7.0 is increasingly basic (alkaline).

phaco- Prefix pertaining to the lens.

phacoemulsification Dissolving the lens by ultrasound.

phacotoxic Intraocular complications due to a diseased lens, such as phacotoxic glaucoma or uveitis, from a leaking hypermature cataract.

phlyctenule Inflamed mass at the limbus, frequently associated with *Staphylococcus* infection or tuberculosis.

photo- Prefix referring to light.

photocoagulation Treatment of retinal vascular conditions, including diabetic retinopathy, with the argon laser instrument.

photophobia Ocular sensitivity or pain when the eye is exposed to light.

photoreceptors Microscopic rod and cone cells of the retina.

phthisis bulbi Shrinkage and atrophy of the eyeball.

pinguecula (plural: pingueculae) Elevated yellowish tissue arising from conjunctiva at the nasal limbus from ultraviolet light or environmental exposure.

pinhole Small opening in ocular occluder through which visual acuity is tested. Improvement of visual acuity with the pinhole test may indicate refractive error or subcapsular cataract. Worsening of vision may indicate corneal opacity or vitreous or retinal disease.

plus lens Convex lens.

posterior capsule Back side of the crystalline lens capsule, which is left in place during extracapsular cataract surgery to support the implanted posterior chamber intraocular lens.

posterior chamber (PC) Intraocular space behind the iris and in front of the vitreous body.

posterior segment The back part of the eye, including the vitreous, retina, optic nerve, and underlying sclera.

posterior synechiae Condition in which the iris adheres to the anterior lens capsule.

posterior uveitis Inflammation of the uvea in the fundus; choroiditis (inflammation of the choroid) involving the overlying retina (chorioretinitis).

preauricular In front of the ear.

precursor That which comes before.

presbyopia Inability to see clearly at close range because of loss of accommodation associated with aging.

prevalence The total number of cases of a disease or condition present at a particular point in time.

primary eye care Component of primary health care that includes promotion of good eye health and treatment and prevention of conditions that can result in blindness.

primary health care worker Health care worker who provides basic health services, including treatment and referral of patients, health education, and promotion of personal hygiene and sanitation.

proliferative diabetic retinopathy Growth of new and abnormal blood vessels in the retina and posterior segment in diabetic patients.

prophylaxis Prevention.

protein-energy malnutrition (PEM) The malnutrition states of marasmus and kwashiorkor occurring together.

pseudophakia Presence of an implanted intraocular lens after cataract extraction.

pterygium Growth on the conjunctiva at the corneal limbus onto the cornea, usually on the nasal aspect.

ptosis Drooping of the upper eyelid.

punctate In a pattern of dots or spots.

punctum (plural: puncta) One of two small openings on the medial eyelids into which tears drain to enter the lacrimal canaliculi.

pupil The round opening in the center of the iris.

purulent Pertaining to or discharging pus.

R

RD Retinal detachment.

RE Right eye.

red reflex Red/orange appearance of the ocular fundus when direct light is shone through the pupil; results from reflection of the vascular choroid (the overlying retina is transparent).

refraction Bending of light rays by a lens; also, the process of determining the refractive error of the eye.

refractive error Optical, non-pathological defect of the eye that prevents light from being brought to a sharp focus on the retina.

retina Light-sensitive tissue lining the inner aspect of the fundus of the eye.

retinal detachment Separation of the sensory layer from the pigment layer of the retina.

retinoblastoma Highly malignant intraocular tumor of early childhood.

retinopathy Disease of the retina. A common retinopathy is from diabetes mellitus.

retinopathy of prematurity Neovascularization of the retina in premature infants secondary to high oxygen levels in the incubator. This was formerly called retrolental fibroplasia (RLF).

retinoscope Instrument used in estimating refractive error by movement of a streak or spot of light across the pupil.

retinoscopy Technique by which refractive error may be objectively measured using trial lenses and a retinoscope.

retrobulbar Behind the eyeball.

river blindness Onchocerciasis.

RLF (retrolental fibroplasia) Former term for retinopathy of prematurity.

rod A type of photoreceptor cell in the retina sensitive to low levels of illumination. The rods serve night vision and motion detection. Compare cone.

S

Schiøtz tonometer A type of indentation tonometer.

Schlemm's canal A tiny circular drainage canal behind the trabecular meshwork in the angle of the anterior chamber.

sclera Tough white fibrous outer coating of the eyeball.

scleritis Inflammation of the sclera.

sclerostomy A surgical opening created under a conjunctival filtering bleb to normalize intraocular pressure in glaucoma.

scrofula A necklace of skin depigmentation and nodular lumps that may occur with tuberculosis.

Seidel test Placement of a small amount of fluorescein on the eye and application of pressure to detect an aqueous leak, usually performed after intraocular surgery when wound leak is suspected.

shortsighted Nearsighted; myopic.

SICS Small-incision cataract surgery.

slit lamp A microscope with a rectangular light source used for close examination of the eye; also called biomicroscope.

Snellen visual acuity chart A card on which are printed optotypes of various sizes according to an international standard; used for measurement of visual acuity.

spring catarrah Vernal keratoconjunctivitis (VKC).

squint British terminology for strabismus.

staphyloma Bulging forward of the cornea and/or sclera due to tissue weakness from malnutrition and/or infection.

stereopsis Binocular depth perception.

sterilization Destruction of microorganisms by means of heat, chemical, or radiation treatment.

steroids Short term for corticosteroids.

stigma A mark or indication.

strabismus Misalignment of the eyes.

stroma Support or foundation layer of a tissue. The corneal stroma is the thickest layer of the cornea.

stye Hordeolum.

subcapsular The inner aspect of the capsule of the crystalline lens. A posterior subcapsular cataract is located in the posterior cortex just beneath the capsule.

subconjunctival Refers to the potential space between the conjunctiva and the sclera.

subluxation Partial dislocation of the crystalline lens.

suture Threadlike material used to make a surgical stitch.

swinging flashlight sign (afferent pupillary test) The 'swinging flashlight' sign; a test with a focal light to determine if posterior segment or optic nerve disease is present. In the affected eye, the pupil may be sluggish to constrict to light and will not constrict further and may even dilate when the stimulus of light in the fellow eye is removed and 'swung' to the affected eye; an important clinical test.

symblepharon Scarring adhesions between bulbar and tarsal conjunctiva.

sympathetic ophthalmia Severe uveitis, often blinding, that occurs in an uninjured eye after injury to the other eye that usually involves injury to the uveal tract.

synechiae See peripheral anterior synechiae and posterior synechiae.

T

tarsal rotation Preferred surgical operation performed on upper eyelid to correct entropion with trichiasis resulting from trachoma.

tarsorrhaphy Surgical joining of the upper and lower eyelids to protect the eyeball.

tarsus (tarsal plate) The fibrous and firm tissue of both upper and lower eyelids that provides form to the eyelids. The tarsal plate is more developed in the upper eyelid.

tears (tear film) Fluid produced by the main lacrimal gland and eyelid glands and conjunctiva that moistens and lubricates the ocular surface.

TEM Traditional eye medications.

temporally In ophthalmology, in the lateral direction; toward the temple.

Tenon's capsule Tissue covering the posterior sclera and extraocular muscles, positioned between the conjunctiva and sclera.

tension (ocular) Intraocular pressure.

tertiary center Comprehensive referral hospital and medical center, often supporting a medical training facility.

TN Tension; intraocular pressure as measured with a tonometer.

tonometry Measurement of intraocular pressure with one of several different precision instruments.

tonopen A portable and handheld instrument for measuring intraocular pressure.

topical Delivery of a medication directly to the surface of the eye or surrounding skin.

torch British usage for hand light or flashlight.

trabecular meshwork Microscopic tissue in the anterior chamber angle through which aqueous fluid drains out of the eye.

trabeculectomy A filtration procedure for glaucoma.

trabeculoplasty Argon laser treatment of the trabecular meshwork to lower intraocular pressure in glaucoma.

trachoma A common ocular infection caused by *Chlamydia trachomatis.* Trachoma is a leading cause of blindness in the developing world.

traditional eye medications Typically, extracts from leaves, herbs, or animal products and often injurious to the eye.

traditional healer Independent and usually non-governmental health care worker trained by apprenticeship in traditional medical practices and beliefs.

traditional medicine Treatment of illness utilizing knowledge, skills, and procedures that follow established practice and are accepted by society.

trauma Injury.

trial lens set A set of individual lenses of various powers used in a trial frame or freely, to determine the appropriate corrective lens.

trichiasis At least one eyelash rubbing on the eyeball or evidence of recent removal of inturned eyelashes. Trichiasis usually occurs with entropion and is a common and frequently blinding complication of trachoma.

U

ultrasound High-frequency sound energy used diagnostically and to emulsify lens cortex in phacoemulsification of cataract.

UNICEF vitamin A capsule Standard dose of 200,000 international units of oily vitamin A; used in mass-dosing children and treating vitamin-A-deficiency conditions.

unilateral One side (of the body) only.

uniocular One eye only.

unplanned ECCE Tearing of the lens capsule, a complication of attempted intra-capsular cataract extraction.

uvea (Latin, 'grape') Ocular tissue that consists of three anatomical parts: the iris; the ciliary body; and the choroid. Sometimes referred to as the *uveal tract*.

uveitis Inflammation of the uvea.

V

VA or **V** Visual acuity.

VAD Visual acuity at distance (6 m or 20 ft).

VAN Visual acuity at near (40 cm or 16 in).

vasoconstriction Narrowing of blood vessels.

VDRL A laboratory serological test for syphilis. (Abbreviation for Venereal Disease Research Laboratory.)

vernal keratoconjunctivitis (VKC) Bilateral severe allergic keratoconjunctivitis that can result in corneal scarring and loss of vision.

VKC Vernal keratoconjunctivitis.

village health worker Primary health care worker living and working in a community or village.

virus (adj. viral) Any of many submicroscopic particles, consisting of genetic material surrounded by a protein coat, that parasitize the cells of living organisms; the cause of a wide variety of infectious diseases, including conjunctivitis and keratitis.

viscoelastic Any of various sterile, thick, fluid substances that are heavier than water and used to maintain the shape of the eyeball and protect the endothelium during intraocular surgery.

visual acuity Degree of sharpness of central (foveal) vision; commonly measured with a Snellen visual acuity card or chart.

visual disability Loss of normal visual acuity resulting in a visual handicap. The World Health Organization classifies all individuals who have a visual acuity of less than 6/18 (20/60) in the better eye as disabled; less than 3/60 (20/400) in the better eye (counting fingers at 3 m) is classified as blindness.

visual field The area within which objects may be seen with one or both eyes.

vitamin A Micronutrient essential for the health of skin, mucous membranes, and eyes that occurs in yellow and dark-green leafy vegetables and in certain animal products such as milk and fish.

vitrectomy Surgical removal of the vitreous from the globe.

vitreous (vitreous body) Clear jellylike substance that fills the part of the eye between the lens and the retina.

W

WHO World Health Organization.

X

xerophthalmia Various changes in the conjunctiva and cornea, including xerosis and Bitot's spots, secondary to vitamin A deficiency.

xerosis Drying and loss of luster of the conjunctiva and cornea in vitamin A deficiency.

Y

YAG laser Short term for Nd:YAG laser.

Z

zonules Fibers connecting the ciliary body to the lens capsule.

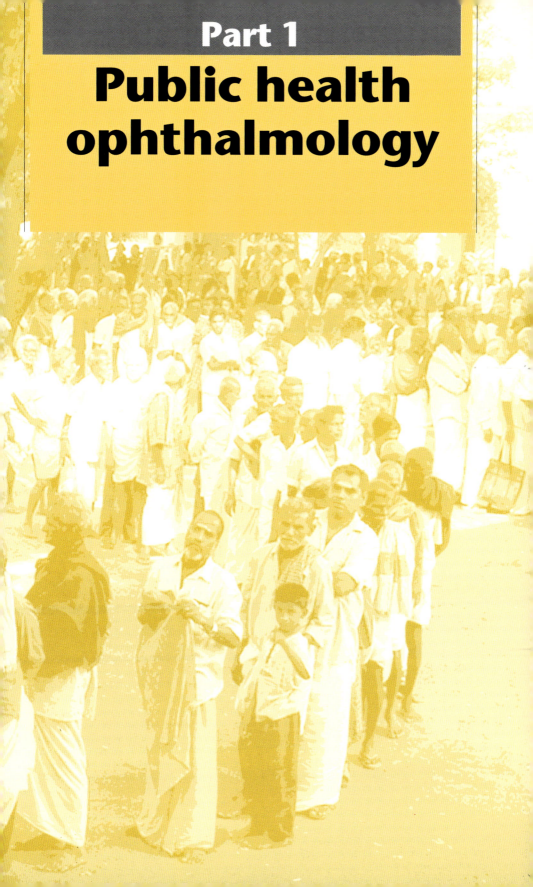

Part 1
Public health ophthalmology

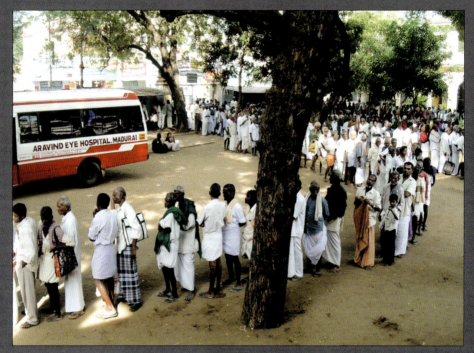

Patients referred to Aravind hospital from outlying communities and transported by bus in community eye care outreach.

1

Public health, preventive care, and eye care delivery

If ophthalmology is our profession, then the prevention of blindness is our business.
Ramachandra Pararagasegaram

An ounce of prevention is worth a pound of cure.
Proverb

You can't plant a seed and expect to pick up the fruit the next morning.
Anonymous

When public health principles are applied to programs for the prevention of blindness, the number of blind individuals in a population or a community can be significantly reduced. Public health programs to control and reduce the rates of blindness are already vitally important for many national eye programs.

Public health differs from curative medicine in several ways:

- The goal of public health is prevention of disease; the goal of curative medicine is treatment and cure.
- The target of public health is a population or community; the target of curative medicine is the single patient.
- The diagnosis of a public health problem is accomplished by a health survey of a population; the diagnosis by curative medicine includes physical examination, laboratory investigations, and other tests.
- Therapy of a public health problem can include health education, improved sanitation and hygiene, and immunization programs; therapy by curative medicine includes drugs and surgery.

- Results of public health are prevention of disease and improvement of quality of life in the whole community; results of curative medicine are limited to individual patients.

Although the predominant focus of this book is to support practical and effective curative medicine in specific situations, there are discussions throughout regarding the appropriate application of public health principles. This chapter, in particular, is specifically devoted to discussion of public health issues in ophthalmology.

Public health ophthalmology

Preventive eye care programs in developing nations teach health care workers to diagnose and treat ocular or systemic diseases or conditions that can cause serious visual disability and blindness if left untreated. The concepts involved in these programs are often amazingly simple; a clean water supply and basic personal hygiene are important to any successful preventive eye care program. In addition to eye care workers, several other types of health practitioners are important in such programs, including integrated primary health care workers, public health nurses, and midwives.

Curative medicine also plays a vital role in reducing blindness rates in developing nations. Cataract, which accounts for almost half of the world's blind, is a surgically curable disease: permanent loss of vision and complications of advanced cataract can be prevented by cataract surgery. Although low vision and blindness from glaucoma cannot be restored, medical and surgical treatment can stop further loss of vision from glaucoma.

The concept of blindness prevention by curative means is exemplified by cataract surgery programs on the Indian subcontinent, where many millions of people are blind from cataract. Many thousands of patients undergo sight-restoring cataract surgery every year through surgical campaigns. These campaigns attract patients who are blind from a variety of causes. All people with eye compaints who attend are carefully screened and diagnosed. Advance publicity ensures large patient attendance for examination and treatment.

Campaigns are often held in remote and underserved areas. Hundreds, even thousands, of cataract operations may be performed during a single campaign.

Indigent patients are provided basic but quality sight-restoring surgery. Eye surgeons volunteer their time and skills, community service organizations provide financial support, and patients learn to fully utilize this unique health service. The surgical cataract campaign is an excellent example of close community cooperation in meeting a public health problem.

Preventive eye care

This section summarizes some of the largest categories of sight-threatening problems facing the developing world (aside from cataract) and possible public health approaches to their effective management. (Defining terminology is given in the respective chapters and the glossary.)

Trachoma

Prevention of blindness in trachoma is possible through early diagnosis and treatment, improved personal hygiene (hand and face washing) (1), and identification of patients with entropion and trichiasis. Corrective eyelid surgery for trichiasis should be performed as soon as possible to prevent further corneal complications. Screening for trachoma can be performed at health stations in villages, at schools, and at prenatal clinics. Particular attention should be paid to children younger than 5 years of age, because they are at high risk of infection in places where trachoma is common. Trachoma control programs involve public health planners, educators, and surgical technicians. Ophthalmologists serve as teachers and perform trichiasis surgery as necessary.

Ophthalmia neonatorum

Prevention of blindness from conjunctivitis of the newborn is achieved by instillation of tetracycline 1% ointment or penicillin drops into the eyes of all newborns. Silver nitrate solution also may be used for pre-

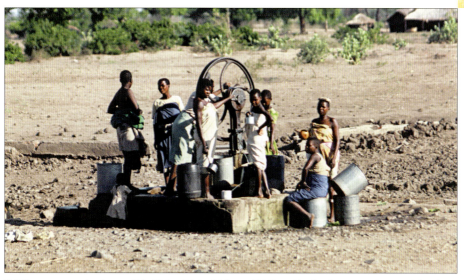

1 Village water point, Lower Shire Valley, Malawi. The availability of fresh, clean water is essential in the control of waterborne communicable disease and trachoma.

vention of neonatal infection. Be aware that a bottle of silver nitrate left sitting at a window in sunlight can evaporate, causing the solution to become more concentrated. Concentrated silver nitrate solution, if applied to the eye, can cause permanent corneal scarring.

If the mother of a newborn is known to be infected with gonorrhea, she should be treated with systemic penicillin in appropriate dosages; her child should be carefully observed for signs of acute conjunctivitis and, if conjunctivitis is present, treated with systemic penicillin and topical penicillin drops. All midwives, nursery attendants, nurses, and doctors should be taught the proper use of tetracycline ointment, penicillin drops, and silver nitrate.

Conjunctivitis and corneal ulcer

Education of the public about the importance of seeking care for a red or painful eye (and avoiding the application of damaging traditional eye medications) is very important in preventing ulceration of the cornea and corneal scarring. An ulcer may follow a seemingly minor injury to the cornea, such as a corneal abrasion. All corneal injuries must be treated promptly to prevent corneal scarring or perforation. All health care workers should understand the importance of early treatment and early referral of an infected eye.

Eye injuries

Ocular trauma and consequent blindness may be prevented by the following means:

- Education programs concerning ocular safety (examples: automobile seat belts to prevent facial and ocular injuries in a collision; avoiding looking directly at the sun or a solar eclipse; using safety goggles while hammering on metal or grinding metal in a machine shop).
- Enforced safety regulations, including protective eye wear, for all workers in industry who are exposed to working conditions where eye injuries are likely to occur.
- Prompt and correct treatment of all eye injuries.

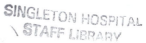

Glaucoma

Prevention of primary open-angle glaucoma, the most common type, is not possible because its cause is not known. Once primary open-angle glaucoma or other glaucoma has been diagnosed, prevention of further loss of vision and blindness is possible by medical and surgical means, as described in Chapter 6.

Early diagnosis and treatment are essential for such a program to be successful. This is a great challenge, because it means examining the entire population. Because glaucoma is more likely to occur after the age of 40 years, screening with tonometry and examination of the optic nerve should be performed on all people aged 40 years and older.

Mass glaucoma screening campaigns can identify new cases needing medical and surgical management. Education of adults about glaucoma can identify further cases; many individuals who could have maintained useful vision if they had been diagnosed and managed earlier appear for treatment of glaucoma at a far advanced stage of the disease. Glaucoma should be suspected in any case of unexplained visual loss.

Primary angle-closure glaucoma cannot be prevented except by providing a surgical iridectomy (removal of a tiny portion of peripheral iris) or iridotomy (making a tiny hole in the iris with a laser), both impractical and expensive to perform on everyone at risk. Angle-closure glaucoma patients undergoing an acute attack have distinct pain and loss of vision; early and correct management of such cases will preserve the eye and vision.

Amblyopia

Prevention of esotropia and exotropia is not possible, but if identified and treated early, visual loss from amblyopia ('lazy eye') resulting from strabismus (squint) may be restored. The earlier the treatment, the better; if a child has not been treated before the age of 6 years, the chance of regaining vision is poor. A high refractive error in only one eye will also cause amblyopia as the patient comes to depend on the other eye. School vision-screening programs can identify children needing attention.

Nutritional blindness

Vitamin A deficiency and malnutrition – marasmus, kwashiorkor, and combined protein-energy malnutrition (PEM) – are major causes of preventable childhood blindness in many nations (Chapter 4). High mortality rates are associated with these conditions; permanent damage occurs in those children who survive. Vitamin A deficiency (xerophthalmia) and keratomalacia should not be considered isolated conditions because they are often only one aspect of generalized malnutrition or starvation.

Several countries (Indonesia and Malawi, for example) have developed national and local programs to address the problem of nutritional low vision and blindness. These programs include surveys to determine the extent of the problem, intervention programs that distribute vitamin A, and programs that improve dietary habits and agricultural practices.

In these and other programs, maintenance dosages of vitamin A are administered to children under 5 years of age; medical assistants trained in recognition of the signs of malnutrition work at the village level to treat and refer patients; and children with malnutrition, diarrhea, and acute febrile illnesses – particularly measles – are treated intensively.

Onchocerciasis

Onchocerciasis ('river blindness') is described in Chapter 9. In Central and West Africa, the disease is responsible for high rates of low vision and blindness.

Blindness from onchocerciasis cannot be reversed. The opportunity to eliminate blindness secondary to onchocerciasis lies in controlling the vector, the Simulium black fly, and thereby controlling transmission of the *Onchocerca* parasite and in the prevention of blindness by community ivermectin chemotherapy treatment.

Corticosteroid use

Corticosteroids, applied topically to the eye in the form of drops or ointment and taken systemically, may have serious ocular side effects. Only one positive effect may result from the use of corticosteroids in ophthalmology, and that is the reduction of external and intraocular inflammation in patients where such drugs are truly indicated, such as in uveitis and post-operative surgical inflammation. Many potentially blinding side effects can result from indiscriminate use of corticosteroids in situations in the developing world where there are few other medical and surgical resources.

Some of these situations, where simple withholding of corticosteroids constitutes preventive care, are described below:

- *Cataract*. Opacity of the posterior area of the lens (posterior subcapsular cataract) can result from prolonged corticosteroid use in any patient, young or old. The cataract does not resolve or disappear when the medication is discontinued. Corticosteroid cataract may be caused by both topical and systemic corticosteroids.

- *Dendritic keratitis* secondary to herpes simplex. This frequently results when corticosteroids are given to patients with red eyes where a diagnosis has not been established. Corticosteroids can cause herpes simplex virus to invade the cornea and can cause the infection to become worse. All patients with external eye infections should be checked with fluorescein dye for corneal herpes simplex infection. *Topical corticosteroids should never be given for a patient with a dendrite corneal staining pattern.*

- *Glaucoma.* Long-term use of corticosteroids can elevate intraocular pressure and cause subsequent glaucomatous optic nerve damage. To prevent loss of vision from this side effect, routine and regular tonometry should be performed on all patients receiving topical or systemic corticosteroids. Discontinuing these drugs will usually allow intraocular pressure to return to normal. If intraocular pressure does not return to normal, the patient should be followed for ocular hypertension and possible glaucoma.

- *Bacterial corneal ulcer.* In general, topical corticosteroids should not be administered to an eye with a bacterial corneal ulcer. The infection can worsen and corneal perforation with loss of the eye may result.

- *Fungal corneal ulcer.* Administration of corticosteroids to a cornea that has sustained an injury with vegetable matter (a wood splinter or rice or maize chaff, for example) may result in a fungal corneal ulceration. Such an ulcer is extremely difficult to treat and frequently results in a blind eye.

- *Corneal abrasion.* Topical corticosteroids should never be used to treat a corneal scratch or abrasion. Bacterial or fungal corneal ulcer can result.

Primary health care and primary eye care

An international meeting of health experts in Alma-Ata in the then-USSR in 1978 outlined a major policy for meeting community health needs. The Alma-Ata declaration (the most recent of its kind) defines primary health care as 'essential health care based on practical, scientifically sound, and socially accept-able methods.' Since the Alma-Ata meeting, greater emphasis has been placed on primary health care program develop-ment.

Primary health care is community based. It is dependent on community involvement and participation. Health care workers, sometimes chosen by communi-ties, serve to promote better living condi-tions and improved health through public health education, teaching good hygiene, and improving waste disposal practices. Primary health care workers also identify and treat common and readily identified diseases and refer patients to health treatment centers.

The principles of prevention of blindness and treatment of common eye diseases – primary eye care – must be incorporated into successful primary health care programs. Primary health care workers can be trained to recognize and manage blinding eye diseases such as cataract, trachoma, and injuries.

Primary eye care includes the following:

- Clinical activities – diagnosis, treatment, or referral of patients with eye disease (**2**).
- Preventive activities – those that prevent blindness, such as routine instillation of tetracycline into the eyes of newborns by traditional birth atten-dants to prevent ophthalmia neo-natorum.
- Promotive activities – education of community leaders, elders, traditional healers, and citizens in the importance of eye care, surgical treatment, and hygiene (**3**).

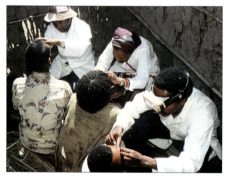

2 Village screening in Ethiopia.

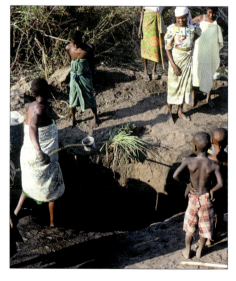

3 Villagers drawing water from an open well in Malawi.

A regular, dependable source of medications and expendable supplies is essential for a successful primary eye care program. Equipment and supplies can be simple, as given below:

- A flashlight (torch) with spare batteries.
- A simplified visual acuity chart.
- Tetracycline 1% eye ointment.
- Vitamin A 200,000 IU capsules.
- Dressings and bandages.

Primary eye care workers require educational support. Their work requires continuous supervision and encouragement by individuals with more comprehensive knowledge and training. Medical assistants, clinical officers, and nurses who have been specially trained in ophthalmology should supervise the primary eye care worker. Training of primary health care workers should include training in basic eye care.

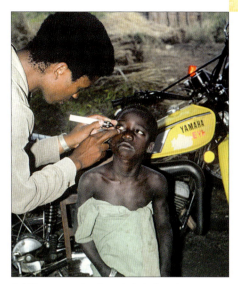

4 Village screening by ophthalmic assistant, Malawi.

A basic curriculum should include the following:

- Testing visual acuity.
- Referring all patients with visual acuity of less than 6/18 (20/60).
- Training in administration of ocular medications.
- Training in application of dressings to the eye.
- Recognizing and managing eye infections.
- Removal of conjunctival and corneal foreign bodies.
- Recognizing and referring serious injuries.
- Promotion of face washing and improved personal hygiene.
- Recognizing xerophthalmia in regions where vitamin A deficiency is a public health problem.
- Carrying out antibiotic prophylaxis of ophthalmia neonatorum.

Health planners can continue to learn from the experiences of new programs in primary health and primary eye care and these experiences and lessons can be helpful in creating effective health programs to improve quality of life. Variations and modifications of these programs are possible. For example, in Malawi, health surveillance assistants from villages – primary health care workers (**4**) – are mobile on motorbikes (donated by a local Rotary Club) to screen patients at the village level for eye disease and to mass-dose all children under age 6 years with vitamin A capsules for xerophthalmia and tetracycline eye ointment for trachoma. The motorbikes (or bicycles) enable them to reach remote villages to screen and treat children and families who do not have access to a health care delivery point.

Organization and delivery of eye care

National eye care programs, where they exist in developing countries, function within government health systems, typically the ministry of health. Many such programs receive assistance from international organizations interested in promoting blindness prevention activities (see Appendix G). A national blindness prevention committee within the ministry of health plans and coordinates activities based on the resources available.

In many developing nations, health services are structured in a multitiered system, as given in the following:

- Community level (in nations or areas of nations where primary health care programs are in place).
- First referral level, usually a health center or district hospital.
- Second referral level, usually a larger hospital, such as a regional, provincial, or state hospital.
- Third referral level, usually the central national hospital and teaching center. If a medical school for training physicians exists, it is usually attached to the third (tertiary) level.

Eye care health workers may be integrated into each level, according to the sophistication of a given country's health services, as follows:

- Community level – a primary health care worker also trained in primary eye care. Referral is to the first level.
- First referral level – ophthalmic medical assistant, ophthalmic clinical officer, ophthalmic dresser, and all ophthalmic auxiliaries trained to diagnose and treat eye diseases common to the region and to do selected surgical operations. Such an eye care worker functions well in a simple but adequate clinic with basic instruments and equipment and inpatient care facilities. In many African countries, many ophthalmic auxiliaries trained at this level are capable of performing ocular surgery, including extraction of an uncomplicated cataract. Referral is to the second level.
- Second referral level – an ophthalmologist at the regional, state, or provincial hospital. Such an ophthalmologist supervises all ophthalmic auxiliaries at the first level in the region. An ophthalmologist based at the second referral level also coordinates and supervises the program for the mobile eye unit, regularly visiting rural health stations with the unit, encouraging and teaching ophthalmic medical auxiliaries and assistants, and performing surgery. Ophthalmic auxiliaries also work at this level and diagnose, treat, and manage inpatients and outpatients. Referral is to the third level.
- Third referral level – the national or central hospital. Here, more sophisticated diagnostic and surgical equipment is available for a wide range of eye surgery. Ophthalmic nurses, ophthalmic auxiliaries, and ophthalmologists staff this health facility. Such a hospital also serves as the training center for ophthalmologists (if attached to a medical school), ophthalmic nurses, and ophthalmic auxiliaries.

Mobile eye units may be based at any level. (For example, motorcycle transport for primary health care workers functions as a 'mobile eye unit' when it delivers primary eye care to communities.) More often, however, mobile eye units are based at the first or second referral level.

The mobile eye unit team may consist of an ophthalmic medical auxiliary, a vehicle driver, and sometimes an assistant (5). The driver may serve as an assistant if a trained assistant is not available. The vehicle is any one appropriate to the environment. A light two-wheel-drive automobile may be sufficient where roads are good; on the other hand, for example in many rural areas where roads may be poorly developed, a durable four-wheel-drive vehicle may be mandatory. The vehicle should not be specially fitted out as an operating theater; such specialized vehicles are expensive and unnecessary. The mobile team visits health facilities in rural areas (6) on a prearranged schedule, examines and treats patients, and performs surgery, including intraocular surgery, according to the qualifications of the eye team.

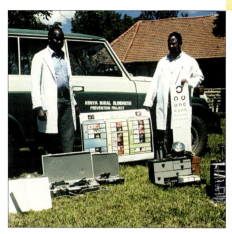

5 Kenya rural eye unit.

A variation of mobile services is that developed by Aravind Hospital in Madurai, India. Here, patients are screened at the village and then surgical candidates are transported to the main surgical center by bus or transportation provided by the hospital. Aravind Hospital systems have been successful in establishing high

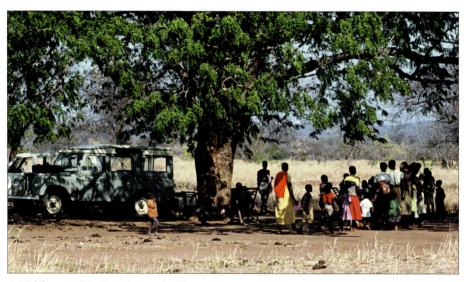

6 Mobile eye unit in Kenya in a rural setting.

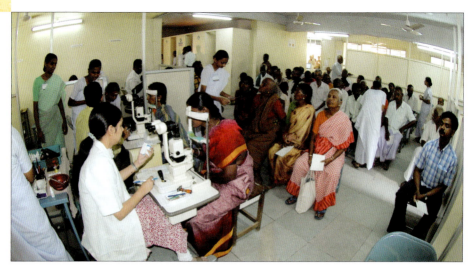

7 High-volume screening clinic, Aravind hospital, Madurai, India.

volume intraocular surgical services using this model (**7**).

Intraocular surgery by non-ophthalmologists

Trained medical auxiliaries perform eye surgery in many African countries. (This is unique to the region, and it is generally not consistent with health care policy in Asia, the Middle East, and Latin America.) These ophthalmic-trained medical auxiliaries extend ocular surgery to rural areas and to patients who otherwise would not be served by an eye surgical team. Many have been trained to do corneal laceration repair and cataract surgery. They also perform eyelid operations (for entropion and trichiasis from trachoma).

Students who are taught intraocular surgery must be chosen carefully. They must be knowledgeable in ophthalmology, interested in surgery, and willing to take on additional responsibility. Previous experience in the operating room is helpful but not necessary. All non-ophthalmologist eye surgeons should be supervised by a well-trained, responsible, and interested ophthalmologist.

The following guidelines are useful (see also Appendix C):

- Students should be naturally skilled in manual tasks (good with their hands).
- They must be able to work with magnification at close range.
- In cataract surgery, students should operate only on patients with uncomplicated cataracts.
- Surgery on one-eyed cataract patients should be performed only by the ophthalmologist.
- All trained eye surgeons should perform surgery on a regular and frequent basis. Non-ophthalmologists should not be trained unless they will be able to perform surgery regularly and frequently.
- Emphasis on concentration and attention to detail in surgical training cannot be overemphasized.

Ophthalmologists, ophthalmic medical assistants, ophthalmic clinical officers, and nurses should be thoroughly familiar with the proper care and storage of instruments. Intraocular surgical instruments are precious; great care in cleaning and storage is necessary, and the instruments must be used only for their intended purpose.

Eye surveys

An efficient and comprehensive national eye care program can be established only if its goals are carefully outlined. In order to establish goals for treatment and prevention of eye disease, the types and extent of eye diseases must be known. Surveys may be necessary to obtain this knowledge in a particular nation or region. After data on blindness and ocular morbidity have been obtained, ministries of health and their blindness prevention committees can make plans for permanent eye clinics, mobile eye units, primary eye care programs, and blindness prevention programs. Public health nurses, ophthalmic medical auxiliaries, epidemiologists, nutritionists, and health planners are all necessary for planning the survey, collecting the data, and analyzing the findings.

Many national and regional eye surveys have been conducted in the past two decades. Some of these surveys have been carried out in Cambodia, India, Indonesia, Kenya, Malawi, Nepal, Saudi Arabia, and other countries. The information gathered from these field studies has been extremely valuable to health planners in those nations and for the broadening of scientific knowledge in ophthalmology generally.

Epidemiological terminology

The language and methods of epidemiology require special study and experience, and are beyond the scope of this book. Two terms that frequently appear in scientific writing require explanation, however, because the term 'incidence' is frequently used incorrectly when 'prevalence' should be used instead.

Incidence refers to the number of new cases of a particular disease that occur over a specified time period, divided by the number of persons at risk. For example, if 45 children with measles appear in a district hospital in a 1-year period, the frequency of measles at that hospital is said to be 45 per annum (per year). If there are 450 children in the district, incidence of measles in the district is 45/450 or 10% per annum.

Prevalence refers to the total number of cases of a particular disease that are present at any one time. It does not refer to the development of new cases over a period of time. For example, if an eye survey reveals 1,000 cases of active trachoma in a district of 10,000 population, the prevalence is 1,000/10,000 or 10%.

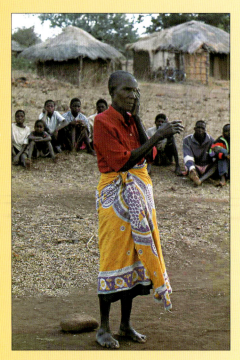

Outreach in Malawi is critical to increasing patient volume. Here, a village elder has her sight tested.

2

Sustainable eye programs

Contributed by Victoria Sheffield, John Barrows,
and Raheem Rahmathullah of the International Eye Foundation

*We can't solve problems by using the same kind of thinking
we used when we created them.*
Albert Einstein

Most developing countries have a national eye care service and many also have private-sector services. Patients obtain eye care either at government hospitals, NGO/missionary hospitals, or private clinics. Private-sector clinics are financially sustainable, but many prefer not to allocate their resources toward care for poor patients. Doctors may 'volunteer' their time in 'charity' hospitals, but they are hesitant to combine a social and private practice simultaneously because they are accustomed to patients either being treated free of charge or paying a fee: they do not have systems in place to accommodate both clienteles. Government and NGO hospitals are dependent on limited health budgets and/or external donations. The situation in many developing countries is that of private services that are prohibitively expensive, serving the upper-income sector of society, or NGO and government services that may be free and serve the very poor and marginalized. There are few services that offer choices for patients who are willing to pay a fee based on a variety of service packages and/or amenities.

General considerations

Providing services to the ever increasing number of visually impaired people involves not only the need to train more ophthalmic professionals, but for existing services to improve quality, become more productive and efficient, and have a variety of services and amenities available to patients at an affordable price. Under-utilization of current services is a challenge.

The major consideration by patients in choosing where to go for eye care is quality. There are two quality indicators, one clinical and the other non-clinical. Clinical quality refers to quality of surgery, post-operative care, and visual outcome. Non-clinical quality relates to the patient's welcome, information provided, addressing of needs, explanation of services and amenities offered, affordable pricing, and courteous behavior during the entire process. It is this quality that drives the demand. There are many examples of patients who choose *not* to access eye care even if it is free, because they know the quality of care is poor. They would seek care in the private sector, however, if they could afford it. The problem, therefore, is the lack of choice in service delivery for patients who have the ability to pay a reasonable fee.

Two major issues to consider are: (1) how to improve the quality of care and service in the government and NGO sectors and (2) how to make the services in the private sector affordable to everyone.

The SightReach® Management program of the International Eye Foundation (IEF) has adapted the Aravind Eye Care System (India) model to Africa, Asia, Latin America, and the Middle East. A key partner in moving this program forward has been the Lions Aravind Institute for Community Ophthalmology (LAICO) in Madurai (India). The IEF invests in eye clinics and hospitals whether they are governmental, public/NGO, or private if they have the leadership, political will, and capacity to change by offering quality care and services at a range of prices attractive to all economic levels of society. These services include not only a sliding fee-scale, but also differing amenities for those who wish to pay for them and creative revenue-generating services that earn income to subsidize services for the poor. In short, the quality of care and surgery is the same for all patients; the differences lie in the choices of amenities and services offered.

An illustration of this principle is that of an airplane. On an airplane journey, all the passengers, whatever the cost of their ticket, arrive at the same destination at the same time. The ticket prices are based on levels of amenity; seating, menu, and so on. Similarly, with eye care, and with cataract surgery specifically, the end result is the same for all patients. All patients receive quality cataract surgery with an intraocular lens (IOL) implanted by a qualified surgeon; the pricing differences lie in the amenities offered. Patients who pay more can make an appointment in the private section, choose their surgeon and the day of surgery, and have a private room. Patients who are subsidized or pay nothing attend the social section, are assigned a physician and surgery time and a shared room or ward, based on the price range the patient chooses. They will have to wait in sometimes crowded waiting areas and will be seen on a first-come-first-served basis.

Sustainability defined

People define sustainability in different ways. Examples include: having a grant to cover ongoing costs for the next 5 years; covering costs entirely from patient revenue; combining income sources to support services. In fact, public and NGO hospitals, and even private hospitals, are never completely financially sustainable; they have grants or special fund-raising campaigns to support special projects. It is also important to recognize that services will not be sustainable unless quality is sustainable. People will not pay for services or donate to services of poor quality. The IEF's definition of sustainability is 'quality eye care services for people at all economic levels that are sustainable through various revenue sources including earned income.'

Increasing the volume of patients while maintaining quality is critical. Fixed costs are recurrent; only variable costs change, so the higher the volume, the lower the unit cost. It is better to have more patients paying a range of prices than just a few paying high prices. The multi-tiered pricing system should be permanent and public, a system in which everyone can see the pricing schedule and make their choice. Zero cost (free) should be one of the options.

The IEF's approach

The following three criteria are critical to success:

- **Leadership**. Change is always a difficult process. To completely transform an eye care service to be more efficient and productive, and to improve quality, staff will have to work in a disciplined manner using standardized procedures. This will make the work more systematic and easier for everyone. There will likely be both internal and external resistance, but the team leader must be committed to the change process.
- **Political will.** There must be a commitment from government and/or governing boards, guaranteeing that an eye clinic will treat both paying and subsidized patients, not just one sector of society.
- **A cohort of paying patients.** There must be enough patients who are willing and able to pay a fee for service as long as there are choices in pricing and a difference in amenities being offered at the various levels.

The patient makes a choice of amenities when seeking quality eye care. The key is to make service choices available.

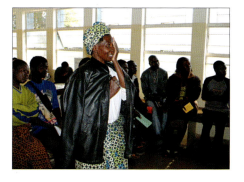

IEF SightReach® Management Program

Instead of investing donor funds to pay for cataract operations or recurring costs that continue to be unproductive, with a Cataract Surgical Rate (CSR) well below recommendations or even the potential of the eye surgeon, the IEF chooses to invest in the changes needed to transform an eye clinic or hospital into a social enterprise serving well-off (paying) and poor (subsidized) patients alike. The focus is to use generated revenue to cover operational costs while donor or other funds are used to increase service delivery to the poor, children, and disabled patients, as well as to fund future expansion for growth (**8**).

In 1999 the IEF began working with government, public/NGO, and private eye clinics, investing to 'fill the gaps.' Each hospital is different, with differing needs to achieve success, but the basic situation and requirements are the same.

Before the implementation of the IEF SightReach® Management Program, the situation was as follows:

Government eye hospitals
- The number of cataract surgeries were below recommended CSR and clinic potential.
- Only the poor and those who could afford private care sought their services.
- No amenities existed to attract paying patients (private clinic, private in-patient rooms).
- No procurement system existed to guarantee availability of consumables as needed.

8 Out-patient walk-in clinic in Lilongwe, Malawi. The Lions SightFirst Eye Hospital in Lilongwe is IEF's first SightReach® Management partner for sustainability planning.

- No control existed over human resources or performance-based evaluations.
- No policies or protocols existed for monitoring improvement.
- Outreach programs existed in only some cases.
- No revenue generating services existed.
- No bank account or accounting policies existed.

NGO/public hospitals

- The number of cataract surgeries was below recommended CSR and clinic potential.
- Fees were usually arbitrary and not related to actual budget.
- Functions were similar to those of a government hospital with little attention to patient service, convenience, and satisfaction.
- Private rooms were often not available for in-patients.
- Policies or protocols were often not in place.
- There was dependence on donor budgets, usually from outside the country.
- Outreach programs were often non-existent.

Private eye hospitals

- The number of cataract surgeries was below recommended CSR and clinic potential.
- Only private patients were seen.
- No multi-tiered pricing system existed.
- No social section with walk-in clinic existed.
- No counselors existed.
- No outreach program existed.
- Usually day care services were offered.
- There were only some rooms for in-patients.
- Often no protocols or policies existed.

After the implementation of the IEF SightReach® Management Program, the following practices were put into effect:

All hospitals

- Assessment of needs to improve quality, efficiency, productivity, and ability to attract a wider range of patients.
- Meetings with stakeholders.
- Hospital team (ophthalmologist, OR nurse, clinic manager, technician) was sent to the Lions Aravind Institute for Community Ophthalmology (LAICO) for their 2-week management course, to see first-hand how a social enterprise functions, and to develop a business plan with follow-up from IEF and LAICO.
- Development and implementation of business plan.
- Establishment of policies and protocols.
- Either initiation or restructuring of the outreach program.
- Establishment of multi-tiered pricing system.
- Establishment of optical services including a workshop with grinding equipment, stocks of frames and lenses, and hire optometrist (9).
- Establishment of bank account and financial policies for handling income.
- Establishment of procurement practices, store room, and employment of procurement manager.
- Hiring and training counselors to meet patient needs at walk-in clinic, answering their questions to alleviate fears, and interfacing with the patient to improve patient acceptance of surgery.

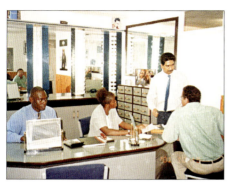

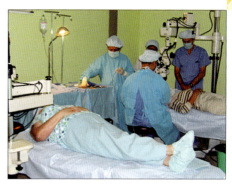

9 An optical service with edging lab at the Lions SightFirst Eye Hospital in Lilongwe, Malawi provides new spectacles at a range of prices and is a major source of revenue.

10 Aravind's operating room assembly-line model was adopted by Visualiza in Guatemala to reduce time between operations.

Government and NGO/public hospitals, additionally

- Hiring of necessary staff, e.g., clinic manager and accountant.
- Establishment of private section and private in-patient rooms to attract paying patients.
- Redesign of patient flow to achieve efficiency (**10**).

Private hospitals, additionally

- Establishment of social section walk-in clinic.
- Establishment of a recovery room for post-operative patients where day surgery is performed.
- Establishment of a ward and/or shared rooms for poor in-patients who require admission.

From 1999 through 2006, IEF partnered with 12 hospitals in eight countries (5 governmental, 4 public/NGO, and 3 private). Their goals were to (1) provide quality eye care, (2) have services and amenities that attract paying patients, (3) have a social section for the poor with services at affordable prices, and (4) use profits to cross-subsidize the cost of care

for poor patients. There was resistance to change as a result of other NGOs raising money to provide only free care. Further resistance came from staff who did not understand what this change was and how it would affect their work, and from the ophthalmology community, which saw NGO services as a threat.

By 2005, the results for seven hospitals in six countries were encouraging. All seven hospitals were practicing modern extra-capsular cataract surgery with an intraocular lens implant (ECCE/IOL). At least one surgeon in all seven hospitals was using the small incision cataract surgery (SICS) technique promoted by IEF. Five of the seven hospitals reported on quality of cataract surgery outcomes using assessment tools developed for this purpose. In addition to numerous other improvements in all hospitals, such as increased staffing and more effective clinical practices, one hospital has introduced and is testing a new patient-management information system.

All hospitals have also established or reorganized outreach campaigns to screen large numbers of persons efficiently, and counsel potential surgical patients to accept surgery at the base hospital. Four of the seven hospitals have established or reorganized optical services for patients, and also the general public, providing refraction and new, high-quality prescription eye glasses at multi-tiered pricing levels.

In terms of efficiency and productivity, in the seven hospitals combined, the number of persons examined increased nearly tenfold between 2001 and 2004. Over this 3-year period there was a 300% increase in the number of patients receiving surgery (of which 70% was cataract surgery). Furthermore, the number of patients treated free or at a subsidized cost increased from 45% in 2001 to 70% in 2004.

It is also noteworthy that, in order to share the successes and tools of the SightReach® program, the IEF supported LAICO's development of a new Internet website called V2020 e-resource (http://www.laico.org/v2020resource/home page.htm), which provides easy access to a large number of documents, articles, manuals, patient-education materials, and new planning tools worldwide.

Finally, the IEF also helped establish LAICO at the Aravind Eye Hospital in Madurai (India) to provide management training for teams from IEF's partner hospitals.

Summary

Ophthalmologists work in differing clinical environments. Each environment has its own challenges, but the potential exists for each to provide quality eye care to wealthy, middle class, and poor patients alike. Government budgets, donor funds, fees, and earned income can be accessed by all sectors and profits can be used to subsidize poor patients. No matter what environment an eye service operates within, if the quality of care is good, its reputation will be good and patients will come for treatment.

Improving the quality of existing services, making them more efficient and productive, and focusing on patient satisfaction, will help to treat the increasing number of visually impaired patients. If eye care services can be accessible, of good quality and affordable, then limited resources can be utilized more efficiently.

There is no single solution to the problem of preventing and alleviating blindness; it has to be a joint effort by governments, NGOs, and the private sector. If quality, accessibility, and affordability are addressed in a coordinated manner, instead of piecemeal, we may be well on our way to meeting the needs of the growing numbers of visually impaired people.

It is recommended that interested persons read the IEF's monograph 'Leading Change – Making Choices' on the website www.iefusa.org.

3

Appropriate technology

Waste not, want not.
Proverb

Use it up; wear it out. Make it do; or do without.
Traditional saying of nineteenth-century German immigrants to United States

A recent trend in health care in industrialized nations has been a shift to and dependence on sophisticated and complicated technological instruments in health care delivery. There is a tendency to rely more on high technology than on basic clinical medical skills for diagnosis and treatment. Commercial ophthalmic equipment and expendable supplies are often scarce or unavailable in developing nations, where monetary resources are usually limited, while the demand for quality eye care services is high.

Technology in health care does not have to be expensive to be effective, and this chapter describes inexpensive but cost-effective technologies in eye care. Appropriate (intermediate) technology in ophthalmology – the local manufacture of cheap but serviceable supplies, and the application of simple, practical ideas – extends basic eye care services even where resources are very limited.

Eye health care workers continuously adapt and revise equipment and supplies to cope with unusual working situations, improvising as they work. The following inventions and ideas are a sample of possibilities that can help eye care services function well in developing nations, often under difficult working circumstances. Eye health care practitioners are encouraged to elaborate on this general approach and to develop and share additional ideas for improved technology in diagnosis, treatment, and surgical programs. The ideas, modifications, and adaptations to eye care technology described in this chapter are presented in three general categories:

- Equipment for ocular examination.
- Instruments and techniques for ocular surgery.
- Expendable ophthalmic supplies.

Equipment for ocular examination

Visual acuity charts

Charts for measuring visual acuity should be made available to district and rural hospitals. It is not necessary to purchase these charts from commercial distributors; inexpensive standard Snellen visual acuity charts can be produced locally. Local printers can print copies of the charts on heavy poster paper or light cardboard for less cost than the commercial variety can be purchased from ophthalmic equipment distributors on plastic boards. Heavy paper or cardboard charts can be mounted on inexpensive thin pressed board; these may be laminated or covered with sheet plastic for protection. *It is very important that the optotypes be reproduced by the printer exactly the same size as they are on the original standard chart.*

An illiterate chart (Landolt C ring chart or Snellen E chart) and either a number chart or a letter chart should be available at health facilities where visual acuity is measured. Such charts can be combined with primary eye care information (**11**).

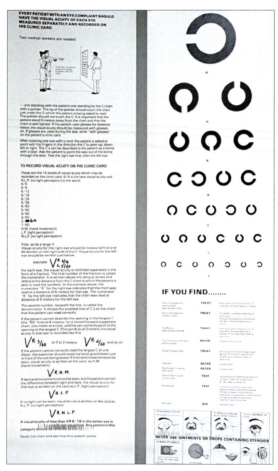

11 Landolt ring C visual acuity chart and instructions for use on reverse side. Developed by the International Eye Foundation.

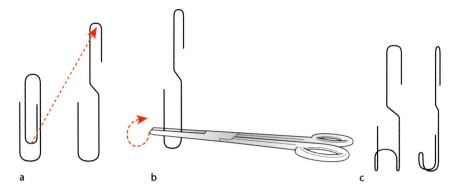

12 Producing an eyelid retractor from a paper clip. Open paper clip (a). Bend larger tip using pliers or hemostat. Finished retractor from front (left) and side (right) (c).

Pinhole

The pinhole test provides valuable information and is part of the routine eye examination. If a pinhole device in a trial lens set is unavailable, a pinhole can be created from a piece of unexposed x-ray film. The film should be opaque, or nearly so. Cut from the film with scissors a circle 5 cm in diameter, with a 2-cm handle. Create a hole with scissors in the center of the circle the size of a pinhead.

Eyelid retractor

High-quality stainless steel eyelid retractors (specula) for adults are very durable and may be sterilized repeatedly and used for years. Commercial pediatric eyelid retractors are manufactured of lighter materials and are often damaged or lost. A metal paper clip or length of heavy spring wire can be fashioned into a substitute eyelid retractor.

To make a paper clip retractor, unfold and flatten the paper clip; then, with a surgical clamp, turn 5 mm of one end of the paper clip back 180° (**12**). This retractor works well either to elevate the upper eyelid or to retract the lower eyelid. Always remember to use topical anesthesia before attempting retraction of the eyelids with any instrument.

Viewing aids

For magnificatiion of the andexae and anterior segment, a hand magnifying lens can be used. A simple biomicrosope (slit lamp) can be fashioned from locally available materials (**13**).

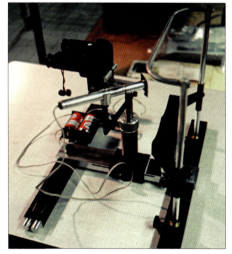

13 A locally made biomicroscope (slit lamp); many disposable articles and some hardware for eye care can be improvised.

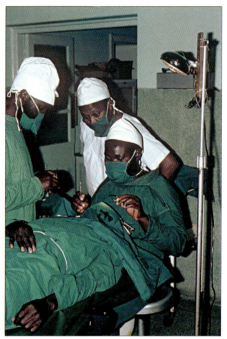

14 Rural eye team in Kenya preparing for surgery using a halogen headlight powered by 12-volt automobile batteries. (Note that surgical gloves were unavailable, as is the case in many rural health care settings. The surgeon and assistant observe stringent asepsis with detailed surgical scrub technique on short, clean fingernails, chemical disinfectant rinse, and strict no-touch surgical technique.)

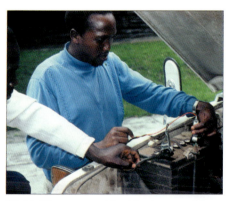

15 Mobile eye team with a 12-volt automobile battery for operating light.

Instruments and techniques for ocular surgery

Portable operating light

An automobile headlight can make an excellent operating light. The halogen headlight is preferable to an incandescent lamp because of greater light intensity. The portable operating room light is convenient in rural areas where electricity is unavailable. It may also be used as a backup light source for eye surgery in communities where electric power is available but shortages are frequent.

A 12-volt automobile battery serves as a power source. The battery and lamp may be taken into the operating room during surgery (14). A disadvantage is the periodic need to recharge the battery; however, if sufficient fuel is available, the battery may be left in a vehicle (a four-wheel drive mobile eye unit operating on a 12-volt electrical system, for example) and a constant charge can be maintained with the engine running (15). The battery leads for the operating lamp are passed into the operating room through a narrow opening of a window.

The halogen lamp can be attached with a small metal hinge to a 10×20×2-cm section of wood with four drilled holes, one in each corner. Sturdy cord passed through these holes and tied to an intravenous pole will attach and elevate the lamp above the surgical field for an excellent surgical light source.

Locally manufactured cryoextractor

A portable and inexpensive cryoextraction unit can be manufactured locally with the help of a machinist (**16**).

The following materials are needed:

- A 2- or 3-liter stainless steel gas canister.
- A one-way gas valve (that fits the gas canister).
- One 20-cm length of copper tubing.
- One disposable cryoprobe.
- A reliable source of liquid freon, nitrogen, or carbon dioxide.

Solder (braise) one end of the copper tubing to the valve outlet, with an adapter if necessary. Load carbon dioxide, nitrogen, or freon in the canister under pressure. An industrial gas supplier can do this. (Industrial gases are available commercially from refrigeration companies and petroleum products distribution centers.) Store the canister in the operating room with the copper tubing attached. A backup full canister should be available.

The disposable cryoprobe handle with tip can be used hundreds of times. Sterilize the disposable cryoprobe handle barrel and tip in surgical spirits (methylated spirits) or in any other suitable chemical disinfectant. Avoid acetone because it will dissolve the plastic handle.

When ready to extract the cataract, the surgeon is handed the cryoprobe handle from the surgical spirits by an assistant. The surgeon dries the handle with gauze or cotton wool. While the surgeon holds the handle, the assistant inserts the copper tubing attached to the canister into the handle. The tubing should reach the closed end of the handle so that gas released through the tubing will cause an ice ball to form on the tip of the cryoprobe (**16**). The assistant opens the valve for 10 seconds, allowing a quantity of liquefied gas to collect in the handle near the tip.

When the ice ball forms, the assistant removes the copper tubing from the cryoprobe. The surgeon then performs cryoextraction. If the ice ball engages the iris or if the surgeon wishes to remove the cryoprobe from the cataract before delivery, the assistant may defrost the cryoprobe tip by drizzling sterile solution from a sterile dropper on the cryoprobe tip. If a cryoprobe barrel handle is unavailable, create one by inserting a 5-mm length of heavy copper wire into the tip of the barrel of a 10-cc syringe. The tip of the syringe that touches the lens capsule should be filed, sanded, and polished smooth.

This system is portable and does not require electrical current as do many standard cryoextraction units. A full 2-liter canister of liquefied gas will provide sufficient gas for 100–150 cataract extractions.

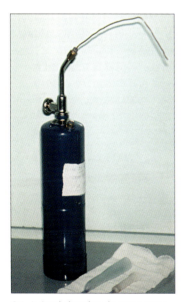

16 A simple handmade cryosystem from locally available canister, copper tubing, resterilizable plastic syringes and industrial inert gas.

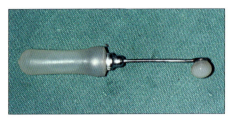

17 Mature cataract with erysiphake: intracapsular cataract surgery is still performed in some rural locations where IOL ECCE/IOL surgery is not feasible or available.

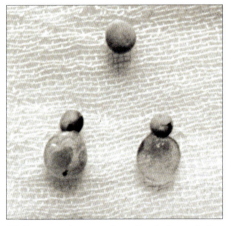

18 Intracapsular extraction using desiccated silica granules in a rural Vietnamese hospital.

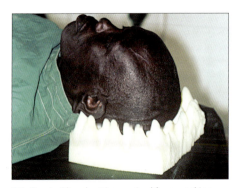

19 Surgical headrest improvised from packing crate insulating material.

Intracapsular cataract extraction without a cryoprobe

The erysiphake and capsule forceps remain valuable tools for ICCE. These instruments can serve as backup to cryosurgery in the event of failure of the cryoextraction system, or either instrument may be used as the primary tool for lens extraction (**17**).

Practice and patience are required to acquire the skills necessary to be effective and safe with the capsule forceps and erysiphake. In experienced hands, both instruments have obvious advantages in rural ophthalmic surgery. They are simple, light, inexpensive, and do not require elaborate backup systems. The rate of capsular tear is lowest with cryoextraction, intermediate with the erysiphake, and highest with capsular forceps.

Desiccated silica granules can be used in intracapsular cataract extraction (**18**). These are the little granules that are contained in the packets of dessicant used to keep humidity low in packaged materials. To use, dry out a granule completely by holding it near (but not in) a flame with a pointed forceps. Then apply the granule to the anterior capsule of the cataract with the forceps. A firm attachment will form, and the cataract can be removed intact by sliding it over the scleral lip. A little counter-pressure at the inferior sclera with a muscle hook can help.

Surgical headrest

Sandbags are frequently used to immobilize the patient's head for ocular surgery. This method is not completely satisfactory. Sandbags are heavy and can fall off the operating table.

A light, one-piece surgical headrest can be fashioned from heavy foam packing crate material or from a portion of a foam mattress. A square of material 25×25x10 cm is needed. Cut away one side of the section and hollow the center out to two-thirds of its depth to accommodate the patient's head. It is not necessary to attach the headrest to the operating table; pressure and friction from the weight of the head will hold it in position (**19**).

Eyelid plate

A metal plate for eyelid surgery provides support and elevation to the eyelid. It also protects the eyeball during surgery.

An ordinary stainless steel soup-spoon handle may be used as an eyelid plate. There is nothing to manufacture because a simple kitchen spoon is all that is required. Insert the tip of the handle under the eyelid. For the assistant, a spoon may be easier to manage than a formal eyelid plate because of its length. Some surgeons find that such a tool offers a more natural operating field for entropion surgery; the spoon handle does not distort the nasal and temporal aspects of the eyelid.

Surgical blades

A razor-blade breaker can be used as an ophthalmic surgical knife. Although this instrument has virtually disappeared in industrialized nations, it remains an inexpensive and efficient tool for many intraocular surgeons in the developing world. One razor blade can provide six surgical knives – three from each edge – of identical sharpness. The cost is only a few cents per knife (**20**).

The best blades for use with the blade breaker are carbon steel blades. Stainless steel blades are more expensive and do not break as easily; they tend to curl when being broken rather than to break clean. Carbon steel blades are *chemically* sterilized (in methyl alcohol, for example) to preserve their sharp edges. *Steam autoclaving and boiling tend to dull blades and sharp instruments.*

Surgical cautery

Electrical cautery systems can fail at inconvenient moments during intraocular surgery. In contrast, the spirit (alcohol) lamp and thermal cautery unit requires only fuel and matches. Such a unit is used as a backup to electrical cautery in some operating theaters; in others, it may be the only cautery available. It is a perfectly reliable source of vascular cautery.

A battery-powered portable cautery is another type that requires a fresh D-cell battery for power. Battery-powered cautery also comes as a disposable microcautery. Intended for one-time use only, the microcautery may be used effectively for ocular surface cautery in up to 20 operations. Chemical and steam sterilization for repeated usage will ruin the disposable unit; the wire tip may instead be sterilized with cotton wool that has been immersed in surgical spirits. In this case, the surgeon holds the contaminated handle with a sterile towel to maintain a sterile field.

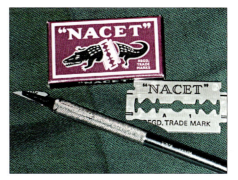

20 A blade breaker provides an inexpensive microsurgical knife for intraocular surgery.

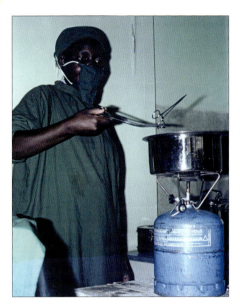

21 Sterilizing large instruments over butane gas stove – not for delicate sharps.

Sterilization

Sterilization of surgical instruments may be difficult in rural hospitals. All ocular surgical instruments must be completely sterile. There is a risk of introducing intraocular infection if sterility is not complete. The methods of sterilization should be simple but effective.

A standard autoclave will serve to sterilize non-precision ocular surgical instruments. If the autoclave is out of order or unavailable, a pressure cooker may be used. Heavier surgical instruments (not sharp instruments or those with fine tolerances), such as mosquito clamps, towel forceps, and large needle holders, may be sterilized in boiling water in a stainless steel cooking pot. Water for boiling and sterilizing instruments must be free of particles. Drip water filters are excellent for removing debris and particles from water to be used for sterilization.

For mobile surgical work, a refillable butane gas stove serves as a good heat source for boiling the pressure cooker or the cooking pot (**21**). It is important to carry two canisters of butane gas so as to always have one as a backup. If autoclave sterilization and butane gas for boiling are both unavailable, an open fire can be used for sterilization boiling. Charcoal is recommended because of its low, intense, and relatively clean flame. Charcoal stoves are available in many country markets in Asia and Africa.

Sterilization of sharp and delicate instruments can be carried out in chemical solutions that are readily commercially available. An effective and inexpensive solution is methylated alcohol (spirits). Methylene blue dye can be added to methyl alcohol to distinguish it from ethyl alcohol and to discourage anyone who might be tempted to drink the alcohol. Instruments to be sterilized are mechanically cleaned with a small brush (a soft toothbrush does nicely) and placed on mesh gauze in a flat stainless steel tray of methyl alcohol an hour before surgery. The instruments are rinsed in hot sterile water after removal from the solution and before placing them on the surgical tray.

Other surgical disinfectant solutions may be substituted for methyl alcohol. Acetone may be used as a surgical disinfectant but it must not be used to sterilize plastic and polymer articles because it will dissolve or destroy these items. Standard surgical blades can be used repeatedly if sterilized properly.

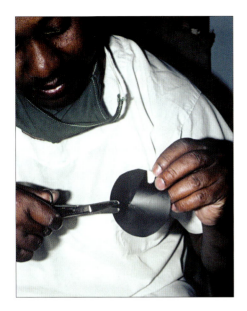

Expendable ophthalmic supplies

Expendable ophthalmic supplies are in constant demand. In many countries, essential items are in short supply.

Protective eye shield

A shield to protect the eye of a postoperative intraocular surgical patient and for perforating eye injuries can be created from discarded X-ray film (**22**), as follows:

- Use a cup or glass as a guide to cut a 6-cm-diameter circle with scissors from X-ray film, heavy paper, or cardboard.
- Make a single scissors cut from the edge to the center.
- Make a pinhole in the center of the circle for pinhole aphakic vision if the shield is for use with a postoperative cataract surgery patient.
- Overlap the cut edges 1 or 2 cm so that a shallow cone is formed. Tape inside and out along the edge.
- Tape the shield securely over the pad that has been placed over the postoperative eye. The pad is removed and only the shield is used after the first postoperative day.

Locally produced ophthalmic medications and spectacles

Imported drugs are expensive and sometimes inappropriate to the actual needs of eye health care workers. Ophthalmic medications can be produced locally for a fraction of the cost of imported versions of the same drugs. They can be constituted from basic ingredients and then packaged or bottled.

Likewise, inexpensive spectacles for indigent patients are always in demand. Spectacles may be produced from basic materials in small optical workshops. Frames may be molded locally and blank spherical lenses edged for framing.

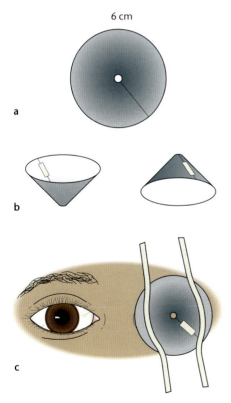

22 Making an eye shield. Cut material as shown (a). Overlap the edges to make a cone, and tape securely (b). Tape over injured eye (c).

Such projects can have the added benefit of employing disabled individuals.

Appendix G (Resource organizations) gives further sources of information on intermediate technology in the local manufacture of spectacles and ocular medications.

Eye pads, surgical sponges, and suture

These supplies need not be purchased commercially. Oval eye pads can be made by first creating a sandwich of cotton wool 1 cm thick between two layers of light muslin gauze. Cotton wool adheres to the gauze. Simply cut out oval eye dressings with scissors from the sandwich.

Cellulose surgical sponges may be cut in 1-cm cubes from long strips. Such sponges are held with small forceps and used in drying the ocular surgical field. This system works better than mesh gauze sponges of the same size, which are not as absorbent.

Individual single needles re-threaded with ophthalmic silk suture from bulk spools may be used as backup if swaged-on ophthalmic suture (commercially fused to the needle) is not available.

Donated supplies

A variety of unused medications, dressings and disposable instruments from ophthalmic sources in wealthy countries can augment eye services in some developing nations. Some supplies, including surgical blades, are used only once and are discarded. These items can be collected from affluent eye clinics and operating theaters and provided to eyecare services in recipient nations, where they can be put to good use after re-sterilization.

Items that can be recycled include the following:

- Fresh, topical ocular medications in quantity that are nearing (but not exceeding) their expiry dates.
- Disposable battery-power cautery units. (These may be used for as many as 20 additional surgical operations.)
- Disposable surgical knives that can be re-sterilized.
- Soft contact lenses of unusual prescription that can be used as corneal splint lenses.
- Packets of sterile gauze or pads that have been opened and partially used. These items can be re-sterilized and safely used in clinics or operating theaters.

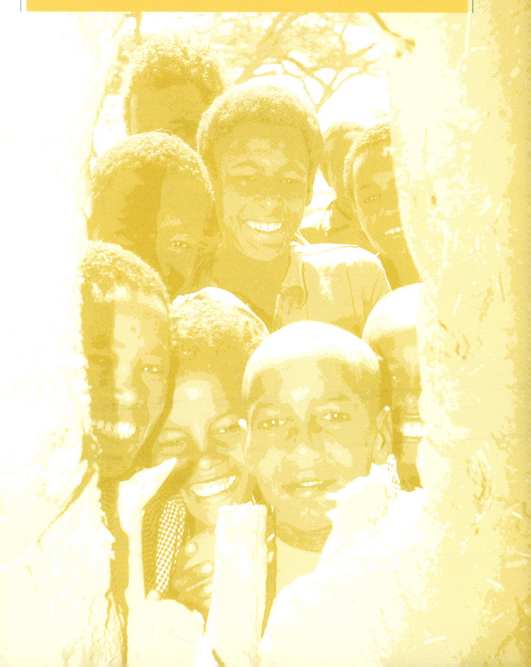

Part 2
Blinding disorders and eye care

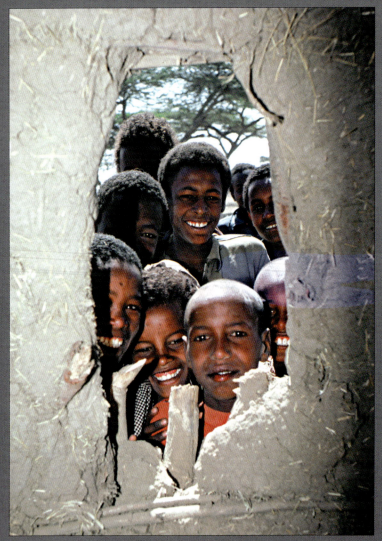

Ethiopian schoolchildren pose for the camera. Ethiopia has one of the highest rates of blindness in the world and the lowest ratio of ophthalmologists (particularly pediatric ophthalmologists) to population.

4

Childhood blindness

...to all those children of the developing world who suffered needlessly until we recognized the source of their tragedy, and who suffer still because governments and the international community have yet to respond in full measure.
Alfred Sommer

Approximately 40,000 children die every day. The majority of these deaths are due to malnutrition, diarrhea, dehydration, and respiratory infection, all preventable or treatable. Most childhood blindness, whether it is from ocular surface infection, malnutrition, trauma, or other less common causes, can also be prevented. Eye health care workers should always be aware of potential blinding or visually disabling consequences of eye disease in children.

Blinding malnutrition

General considerations

Childhood malnutrition, combined with external ocular infection and inflammation, takes a tragic toll on human eyesight. These preventable blinding conditions are easily diagnosed and treated. The key aspect of malnutrition that affects the metabolism of the eyes is vitamin A deficiency.

Vitamin A is necessary for growth, health, and proper functioning of surface tissues, including the epithelium of skin and mucous membranes, and of ocular tissues, specifically the cornea, conjunctiva, and retina. An adequate dietary intake of vitamin A will maintain the normal functioning of the cornea and retina.

Vitamin A occurs naturally (precursors) in dark-green leafy vegetables, and in yellow vegetables, tubers, and fruits; and occurs (preformed) in eggs, milk, liver, and fish. In regions of the world where vitamin A deficiency is a public health problem, most dietary intake of vitamin A is from dark-green leafy vegetables and yellow fruits and vegetables.

Vitamin A is fat soluble. To be absorbed into the body, it binds to a specific protein in the intestine. It is then transported in the bloodstream to the liver where it is stored. When the dietary intake is not sufficient to meet the body's needs, stored vitamin A is released from the liver for use by body tissues. When liver stores are exhausted, vitamin A deficiency results and surface epithelial tissues become abnormal.

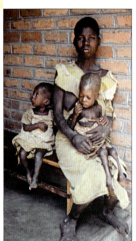

23 Mozambican refugee mother with children with severe protein-energy malnutrition (PEM).

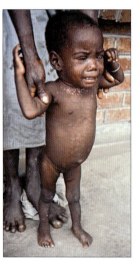

24 Child with severe protein-energy malnutrition (PEM). The child is disabled by night blindness, xerosis, Bitot's spots and trachoma.

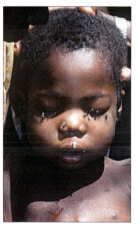

25 Kwashiorkor/marasmus (protein-energy malnutrition); the child has night blindness, xerosis, and Bitot's spots.

Xerophthalmia is a term that describes the ocular changes resulting from vitamin A deficiency. Xerosis means drying of the conjunctiva and corneal epithelium. While conjunctival xerosis may signal mild vitamin A deficiency, corneal xerosis indicates more severe deficiency. Children with corneal xerosis are likely to suffer from systemic illnesses, including diarrhea, respiratory illnesses (pneumonitis and pneumonia), and measles.

Keratomalacia (softening and melting of the cornea) is the most severe ocular form of vitamin A deficiency. Keratomalacia destroys the cornea and permanent blindness usually results. It occurs with acute, severe deficiency of vitamin A. The presence of keratomalacia indicates a poor prognosis for health and life; more than 50% of children with keratomalacia die because of associated poor nutritional status and susceptibility to disease.

The generalized starvation syndromes marasmus (calorie deficiency) and kwashiorkor (protein deficiency) usually do not occur separately; the term protein-energy malnutrition (PEM) indicates that both calorie and protein deficiency are present (**23–26**). These starvation syndromes have high mortality rates. Keratomalacia occurs in starvation syndromes when vitamin A (and other essential vitamins) are deficient. Measles is also frequently associated with malnutrition.

Even mild vitamin A deficiency is associated with reduced survival in early childhood. Children under age 5 years and infants who are vitamin A deficient are at risk of developing life-threatening diarrhea and respiratory infections.

Severe xerophthalmia should not be considered an isolated ocular disease because it usually occurs with generalized malnutrition or starvation. Keratomalacia and corneal xerosis are both ocular and medical emergencies and treatment should always include nutritional rehabilitation.

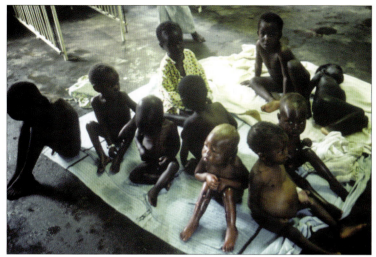

26 Nutrition rehabilitation ward. Children with marasmus and kwashiorkor are at risk of xerophthalmia and kerato-malacia.

Diagnosis and management history

Failure to see adequately in dim light (night blindness or *nyctalopia*) is a classic symptom of chronic vitamin A deficiency, and questions about poor vision at night should be asked of parents or guardians when taking the ocular history in order to diagnose vitamin A deficiency. Parents will report that their children have difficulty moving about the house in the evening and at dusk. Usually there is a specific term in the local language for night blindness in communities where vitamin A deficiency occurs. A careful dietary history with specific questions about the consumption of dark-green leafy vegetables, yellow vegetables and fruits, and milk and eggs will assist in establishing the diagnosis of vitamin A deficiency.

Signs of vitamin A deficiency

Thinning and lightening of hair, weight loss, and drying and scaling of skin are signs of systemic malnutrition. The WHO classification of xerophthalmia is shown in *Table 1*.

Table 1	**Xerophthalmia classification***
XN	Night blindness
X1A	Conjunctival xerosis
X1B	Bitot's spot
X2	Corneal xerosis
X3A	Corneal ulceration/keratomalacia involving less than one third of the corneal surface
X3B	Corneal ulceration/keratomalacia involving one third or more of the corneal surface
XS	Corneal scars presumed secondary to xerophthalmia
XF	Xerophthalmic fundus

*This table displays the World Health Organization's formal categorization.

The following notes provide annotation and explanation of the ocular signs found:

- **X1A** The conjunctiva has a rough, dry appearance in xerosis.
- **X1B** Bitot's spot is a whitish, slightly elevated, foamy spot on the temporal conjunctiva. It overlies conjunctival xerosis and is usually bilateral. It is characteristic of chronic vitamin A deficiency (**27, 28**).
- **X2** Xerosis causes the cornea to lose its bright, lustrous appearance. Light from a flashlight (torch) reflected from a xerotic cornea appears diffuse, scattered, and dull (**29**).
- **X3A** Corneal ulcer is a defect that may penetrate and perforate the cornea, leaving it permanently damaged. Corneal ulceration often occurs with corneal xerosis.
- **X3B** In keratomalacia, the cornea becomes soft and appears to melt (**30**). The corneal surface is irregular. Corneal clouding (secondary to edema) is present. Secondary bacterial infection can occur.
- **XF** An accurate history of night blindness indicates that retinal changes of vitamin A deficiency are present.

Treatment and prevention
Vitamin A deficiency is not an isolated syndrome but is dependent on many dietary, economic, and social factors. The solution should involve nutritionists, ophthalmic health workers, and health planners. It is important that local community individuals be involved and educated in health and nutrition. This should include workers in a position to plan the types of agricultural plantings.

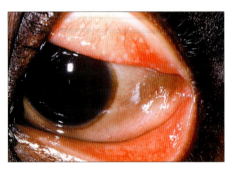

27 Bitot's spot and active trachoma.

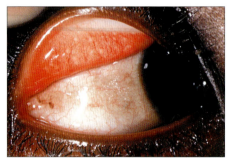

28 Bitot's spot, xerophthalmia, and active trachoma.

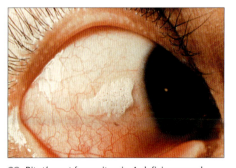

29 Bitot's spot from vitamin A deficiency and xerophthalmia.

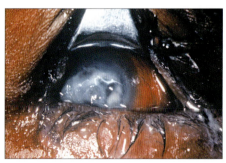

30 Keratomalacia.

Table 2 Xerophthalmia treatment schedule for children between 1 and 6 years old

Immediately on diagnosis	200,000 IU of vitamin A orally*
Following day	200,000 IU of vitamin A orally
4 weeks later	200,000 IU of vitamin A orally

*If there is persistent vomiting or profuse diarrhea, an intramuscular injection of 100,000 IU of water-soluble vitamin A (but not an oil-based preparation) may be substituted for the first dose. (The use of sterile syringes and needles is, of course, essential.)

Table 3 Disease-targeted prevention schedule for preschool children at high risk* †

Children over 1 year and under 6 years old	200,000 IU of vitamin A orally at time of first contact with health care worker for each episode of illness
Infants under 1 year old and children of any age who weigh less than 8 kg	100,000 IU of vitamin A orally at time of first contact with health care worker for each episode of illness

*For example, those presenting at a health center with measles, severe protein-energy malnutrition, acute or prolonged diarrhea, or acute lower respiratory infections. (In areas where measles is a particularly severe disease, with a high mortality and a high risk of blindness, as in Africa, it is appropriate to use the full treatment for xerophthalmia as described in Table 3.)

†This dose should not be given to children who have already received a high-dose vitamin A supplement within the preceding month.

Table 4 Universal-distribution prevention schedule for preschool children and lactating mothers

Children over 1 year and under 6 years old who weigh 8 kg or more	200,000 IU of vitamin A orally every 3–4 months
Children over 1 year and under 6 years old who weigh less than 8 kg	100,000 IU of vitamin A orally every 3–4 months
Infants	100,000 IU of vitamin A orally at 6 months*
Lactating mothers	200,000 IU of vitamin A orally at delivery or during the next 2 months; this will raise the concentration of vitamin A in the breast milk and so help to protect the breast-fed infant

*Best treatment protocol: 25,000 IU of vitamin A orally at each of the three diphtheria–pertussis–tetanus visits, the polio immunization, and then at 9 months (measles immunization).

Breast feeding is strongly recommended for newborns and infants, and mothers should be encouraged to continue breast feeding through the first 2 years of a child's life. Dark-green leafy and yellow vegetables, rich in the precursors of vitamin A, should be included in the diet whenever available. Adequate fat and protein in the diet are also needed to improve absorption and utilization of vitamin A.

Direct distribution of vitamin A in the form of capsules is an emergency measure needed in many areas of the developing world. The treatment schedules in *Tables 2–4* show current World Health Organization recommendations.

Corneal scarring from vitamin A deficiency

A xerotic (dry) corneal epithelium is susceptible to infection by bacteria, herpes simplex virus, measles virus, and fungi. A corneal ulcer from these agents will likely result in scarring. Visual acuity may be markedly affected. Corneal ulcer can perforate the cornea, allowing the iris to prolapse through the cornea (**31**).

With weakening of the corneal tissue, the thinning cornea can also bulge forward, producing a staphyloma (**32**). The eye can shrink and atrophy (phthisis bulbi) from perforation of the cornea and from infection. Children with keratomalacia should always be hospitalized. Intensive nutritional rehabilitation is essential to save the child's life. Even if a child survives acute starvation with keratomalacia, his or her eyes are frequently blind from scarring or infection.

Measles and childhood blindness

Measles is an acute febrile childhood viral illness that is commonly associated with vitamin A deficiency and malnutrition. It occurs worldwide, but in many industrialized countries epidemics of measles have been controlled by vaccination programs. Measles remains a problem in many developing nations in Africa and Asia. It is a major cause of childhood mortality and blindness, particularly in Africa. A West African proverb states, 'Don't count your children until after measles.' Measles can be seasonal and epidemic and is highly contagious.

The measles virus infects epithelial surfaces: skin, mucous membranes, conjunctiva, and the corneal epithelium. Measles and other febrile illnesses depress

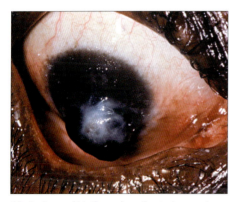

31 Prolapse of iris through perforated corneal ulcer. Scarring (fibrosis) over the prolapsed iris has occurred.

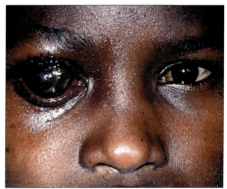

32 Anterior staphyloma involving the entire cornea in a child with vitamin A deficiency.

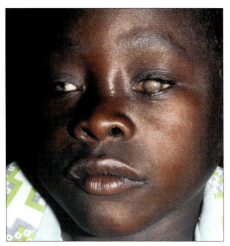

33 A child with corneal scarring, who survived vitamin A deficiency and measles.

liver stores of vitamin A and serum protein, worsening the child's nutritional status. Xerophthalmia, corneal ulcer, and keratomalacia may appear in malnourished or starving children with the onset of, or during the course of, measles. Even if the child survives measles, corneal scarring or phthisis bulbi in one or both eyes can result (**33**). Measles contributes significantly not only to childhood mortality in developing nations but also to childhood blindness.

In regions of the world where trachoma is endemic, it also contributes to blindness from measles and xerophthalmia. Trachoma and measles both attack the conjunctival and corneal epithelium.

Prevention of blindness from measles
Low vision and blindness from measles that occurs with vitamin A malnutrition can be prevented. Early case identification, accurate diagnosis, and proper management are essential, along with comprehensive vaccination programs.

An undernourished child with measles is a medical and ocular emergency.

The child should be hospitalized and medical and nutritional rehabilitation begun. Vitamin A supplementation according to the age of the undernourished child (*Table 2* and *3*) should be administered. In addition, tetracycline 1% ointment should be applied every 12 hours to both eyes for as long as the fever and skin changes of measles persist. Tetracycline antibiotic ointment not only prevents secondary bacterial infection but also moistens the xerotic epithelium of the ocular surface.

Daily examination of both eyes is necessary. Look for corneal ulceration, bacterial conjunctivitis, and xerophthalmia. Corneal ulceration and bacterial conjunctivitis should be managed according to the principles outlined in Chapter 11.

A widely available and highly effective vaccine prevents measles in children. Ideally, all infants should be vaccinated against measles at 9 months of age. Vaccination has been a major factor in controlling measles in many countries; the vaccine is now reaching more than 50% of children worldwide.

The vaccine requires refrigeration and an effective cold chain. Maintaining the cold chain is a challenge in many countries. Nevertheless, population coverage levels with measles vaccine are increasing rapidly, especially in Africa. A vaccine that could be developed would make possible the prevention of measles blindness.

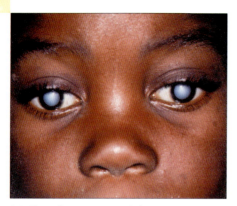

34 Bilateral mature congenital cataracts. Compare with 35, right.

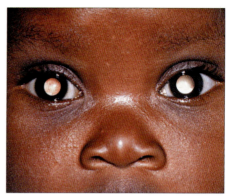

35 Bilateral retinoblastoma. This presentation should never be confused with bilateral congenital cataracts in a child.

Congenital cataract

Although rare, congenital cataract should be suspected when a child with subnormal vision is identified. It is usually bilateral, and can present with bilateral white pupils (**34**). Early surgery is necessary, and the child should be referred as soon as possible. Included in the differential diagnosis of leucocoria in children is retinoblastoma (see **35**).

Retinoblastoma

This is a rare but highly malignant tumor of the retina in children (**35**). Retinoblastoma usually develops before the age of 3 years, but it may present later in childhood. Sudden onset of strabismus can be an early sign. The tumor most frequently is unilateral, but it can be bilateral. Retinoblastoma may cause pupillary abnormalities (unequal size of pupils and unequal or no reaction to light stimulus in the affected eye). If the tumor blocks the visual axis and macula, visual acuity will be affected. Advanced retinoblastoma can cause leucocoria and must be distinguished from other causes of white pupil (see **34** – congenital cataract).

Retinopathy of prematurity

Retinopathy of prematurity (previously called retrolental fibroplasia) occurs in premature infants of low birth weight that have been treated with supplemental oxygen in incubators. High oxygen levels apparently stimulate new vessel growth (neovascularization) in the incompletely formed retina of the premature infant. The result can be, with time, proliferative retinopathy and retina detachment resulting in blindness. The eye health care worker ensures proper examination of the ocular fundi of all premature infants who have received supplemental oxygen in the hospital.

Congenital glaucoma

This condition require early treatment by surgical specialists to conserve vision in infants and children. Always suspect congenital glaucoma in a newborn or infant if the corneae appear to be larger than normal (**36**). In infancy, congenital glaucoma may also present with excessive tearing and eyes that appear to bulge.

Conjunctivitis in newborns

Conjunctivitis of the newborn can be caused by one or several bacterial agents contracted at the time of birth from the mother's birth canal. The most destructive is gonococcal conjunctivitis (keratoconjunctivitis if both the conjunctiva and cornea are involved) and should be treated immediately to prevent serious damage (**37**). Please refer to Chapter 1 (Public health), page 36 and Chapter 11 (External disease), page 155, for management.

HIV/AIDS and malaria

Other infectious diseases also impact on children's eye health. HIV/AIDS may present as uveitis or herpes zoster (see Chapter 12, page 174). Eye findings in malaria may occur in the retinal vasculature and require papillary dilation and good ophthalmoscopy to diagnose. Malaria and HIV/AIDS also contribute to childhood mortality.

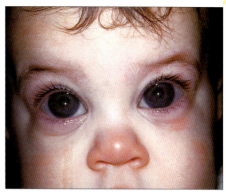

36 Congenital glaucoma. Note bilaterally large corneas.

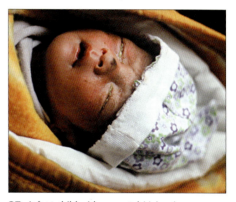

37 Infant child with neonatal *Neisseria gonorrhoeae* keratoconjunctivitis.

Screening of children

All children with strabismus (squint; see Chapter 12, page 170) should be properly evaluated and operated on by a specialist as soon as possible. Screening of school children can be performed by mobile eye services rather than performing examinations in clinical settings. An assessment of visual acuity should be performed on all children if possible in screening campaigns. Children with strabismus, leucocoria, ptosis, or skin lesions of the ocular adnexae should be examined by the specialist if the diagnosis is not obvious.

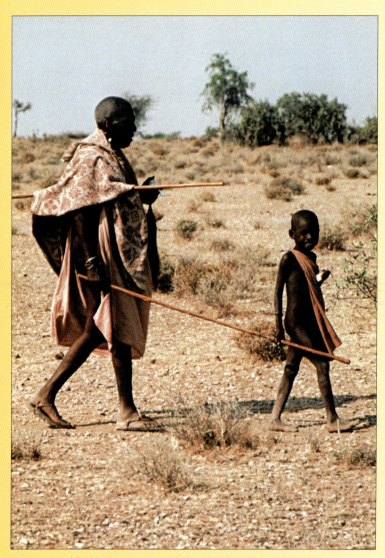

Kenyan man, blind from cataract, guided by grandson with stick.

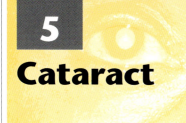

5

Cataract

One of the basic human rights is the right to see.
Statement from the Central Council for Health, New Delhi, India, 1976

Cataract is the most common – and fortunately one of the most easily remedied – cause of visual incapacity and blindness.
Sir Stewart Duke-Elder

Gentle handling of the tissue, understanding its nature, precise movements and right judgment at the right time produce good results. The reward is seen the next day on the happy face of a person whose sight is restored.
Chundak Tenzing, Medical Director, Seva Foundation

Cataract is the leading cause of blindness and low vision in the world. Most cataract blindness is found in the developing world. Although the vast majority of cataracts cannot be prevented, cataract is surgically curable. Inexpensive and efficient surgery can reduce the large number of people blind from cataract. Cataract surgery is one of the most cost-effective public health interventions worldwide. The effort to reduce the number of patients blind from cataract through improved ocular surgery delivery to disadvantaged populations and to determine through research how to prevent or delay the onset of cataract are two of the major public health challenges of our time.

Epidemiology

Approximately 18 million people are blind from cataract (visual acuity less than 3/60 [20/400]). In most countries of Africa and Asia, cataract accounts for approximately half of all blindness. Approximately 60 million more are visually disabled by cataract (visual acuity better than 3/60 but worse than 6/18). An estimated 1.25 million additional people are blinded or visually disabled by cataract annually (global incidence).

The majority of those blind from cataract live in developing nations. Poverty contributes to high cataract rates because poor people do not have easy access to health care and eye care. In industrialized nations where health care systems are highly developed, cataract is diagnosed and usually operated on when it interferes with the patient's ability to function.

Although cataract can occur at any age, most cataracts are related to aging. The majority of cataract-related blindness and visual disability occurs after 50 years of age. It is estimated that by the year 2020, there will be 1.2 billion people aged 60 years and older, and three quarters of them will live in developing nations. As the global population grows and ages, the incidence of cataract will increase.

The economic loss due to blindness and visual disability from cataract is enormous. Blind people are unable to work and able-bodied people are required to care for them. Data from India indicate that economic loss from cataract in that country is approximately US$2 billion annually. Economic loss from cataract blindness on a global scale is unknown.

Definition and etiology

Cataract is defined as any opacity of the natural crystalline lens. The term cataract is derived from a Greek and Latin word meaning 'to fall down' or 'waterfall.' Early medical practitioners believed that something had fallen in or behind the eye. Cataract causes blindness and visual loss not only in human beings, but also in other mammals and birds.

Most lens opacities are small and do not interfere significantly with visual acuity. Visual loss from cataract, other than cataract resulting from trauma, is gradual, progressive, and painless.

Aphakia is the condition of the eye without a lens. An eye that has undergone surgical removal of a cataractous lens is aphakic. An eye that has had surgical removal of a cataractous lens with implantation of an artificial intraocular lens (IOL) is *pseudophakic*.

The etiology (cause) of cataract may include any of the following:

- Injury, or trauma, to the lens. Penetration of the lens by a foreign body usually results in cataract. A contusion injury to the eyeball without penetration may also produce cataract. Injury is a major cause of secondary cataract.
- Inflammation within the eye (usually uveitis).
- Metabolic conditions; diabetes mellitus is the most common.
- Other intraocular disease, including retinal detachment and, rarely, intraocular tumors (melanoma and retinoblastoma).
- Congenital cataract, a rare condition in children, may occur at birth or develop in early infancy. A familial tendency may cause early development of cataract in childhood or early adulthood.

Other, less certain, etiological factors (not absolutely proven) may be associated with cataract:

- Excessive exposure to sunlight (especially the ultraviolet radiation in sunlight) in tropical countries may be one reason for the high rate of cataract in the tropics.
- Poor nutrition in developing countries may contribute to the development of early cataract in some people.
- Acute diarrhea in early life may be associated with cataract development.
- Smoking is almost certainly related to the early development of cataract.
- Commonly used drugs may lead to early onset of cataract. Prolonged use of corticosteroids in particular, both topical to the eye and systemic, can cause cataract.

Anatomy of the crystalline lens

The human lens is composed of four basic structures (**38**):

- The *capsule*, the elastic clear membrane enclosing the lens.
- The *epithelium*, a layer of cells lying beneath the anterior lens capsule.
- The *cortex*, clear protein material forming the bulk of the lens and surrounded by the lens capsule.
- The *nucleus*, or center of the lens, which is soft in infancy and childhood and becomes progressively harder with age.

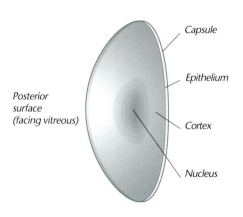

Capsule

Epithelium

Posterior surface (facing vitreous)

Cortex

Nucleus

38 Anatomy of the crystalline lens.

Classification

There are numerous ways that cataracts are classified; some of these categories (and terms within categories) overlap.

Cataract may be classified according to *age of patient at onset*:

- Infantile cataract.
- Developmental cataract (familial, developing in childhood or early adulthood).
- Adult-onset cataract (age-related cataract); by far the largest group, sometimes called 'senile' cataract.

Cataract may be classified according to the following *etiology*:

- Congenital cataract, due to an inherited tendency or secondary to maternal origin such as in syphilis or rubella.
- Traumatic cataract (injury).
- Metabolic cataract (secondary to diabetes or other systemic disease).
- Secondary cataract, due to uveitis and intraocular infection or due to excessive use of corticosteroids.
- Uncomplicated cataract (no known cause).
- Complicated cataract. This is a collective term for cataract secondary to a known condition such as trauma, uveitis, or diabetes.

Cataract may be classified according to the following *anatomy*:

- Nuclear cataract. This is hardening of the nucleus with age.
- Cortical cataract. The cortex becomes cloudy, usually with age.
- Cortical–nuclear cataract (cataract of both the nucleus and the cortex).
- Subcapsular cataract (opacity of the capsule on its inner surface). Excessive use of corticosteroids can cause posterior subcapsular cataract at any age.

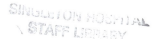

Cataract may be classified according to the *density* of the cataract:

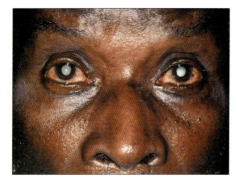

39 When visual acuity cannot be obtained because of density of cataracts, check pupillary reaction. If the pupils react normally to focal light stimulation, cataract surgery should be undertaken.

- ■ Incipient cataract. This early lens opacity may cause little or no decrease of visual acuity.
- ■ Immature cataract. A lens opacity is present and causes minor disturbance in vision.
- ■ Mature cataract. The lens appears whitish or milky and vision is greatly affected (**39, 40, 41**).
- ■ Intumescent cataract. The lens is milky and swollen.
- ■ Hypermature cataract. The appearance of the lens in the pupil is completely white, and the lens is shrunken (**42**).
- ■ Morgagnian cataract. The cortex has liquefied and support for the hard nucleus is lost. The nucleus floats in the fluid cortex within the capsule (**43**).

40 A 45-year-old man with pellagra; his poor nutritional status could have contributed to the early development of bilateral mature cataracts.

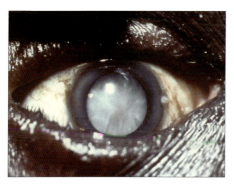

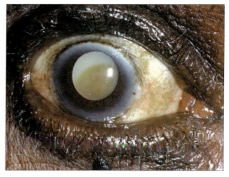

42 Bilateral mature cataract patient's first presentation at clinic.

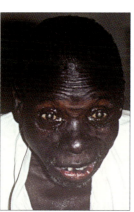

41 Mature cortico-nuclear cataract.

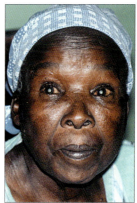

43 Morgagnian cataract with liquefied cortex.

Cataract may be classified according to *location*, as follows:

- Luxated, or dislocated (completely out of position) (**44**).
- Subluxated (partly out of position).

Prevention

The vast majority of cataracts cannot be prevented; however, visual disability and blindness from some types of cataract can be prevented, as stated below:

- Secondary traumatic cataract in children can be prevented by education and eye safety.
- Safety measures (such as protective spectacles or goggles for workers in certain industrial occupations) can prevent traumatic injuries that can cause cataract.
- Early detection and treatment of uveitis can prevent blindness from secondary cataract.
- Prompt treatment of penetrating eye injuries can prevent secondary cataract.
- Careful monitoring of patients on medications that are known to cause cataract (such as corticosteroids) can prevent posterior subcapsular cataract.
- Proper control of diabetes mellitus may delay the onset and progression of metabolic cataract.

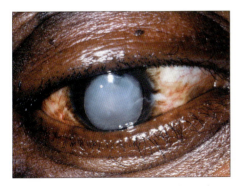

44 Mature cataract spontaneously dislocated into anterior chamber.

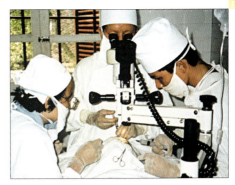

45 Intraocular microsurgery at a rural hospital in Nepal.

Surgical management

Surgical removal of the cataractous lens and replacement of the optical power of the lens is the only effective method to restore vision lost as a result of cataract. Many different cataract procedures are currently in use. This chapter will consider in depth both intracapsular cataract extraction (ICCE) and extracapsular cataract extraction with intraocular lens implantation (ECCE/IOL) which can be performed, with appropriate time-saving techniques, in 15 minutes or less in optimal conditions by an experienceed surgeon (**45**).

Cataract extraction is one of the most commonly performed operations in all of surgery. It is a very successful operation. Studies have shown that 95% of patients operated on for cataract have their visual acuity improved at least two lines on the visual acuity chart. On this basis, 95% of all cataract surgery is successful.

In contrast, there is no effective medical treatment for cataract; that is to say, there is no medication or drug presently known that will prevent or delay the onset of cataract. It is possible that research may eventually provide the knowledge and medical means to prevent cataract.

General considerations

Cataract surgery was performed by medical practitioners of ancient civilizations. Susruta, the legendary Indian surgeon, described the condition of cataract and an elementary form of cataract surgery more than 2,000 years ago.

Couching is an ancient technique, still in practice, of dislocating the cataract posteriorly into the vitreous. It is accomplished by inserting a blunt needle into the eye at the limbus or by the application of continuous external pressure at the limbus, which ruptures the zonular attachments of the ciliary body to the lens. Couching is practiced by traditional healers in several regions of the world, mainly in Asia and Africa. It is not an acceptable substitute for surgical cataract extraction because of its high complication rate. Couching results in many blind eyes from complications.

Modern cataract surgery in wealthy industrialized countries is expensive due to the high costs of staffing and the sophisticated instrumentation and high technology. It is not economical to apply these advanced surgical systems to the tremendous number of cataract patients in developing countries. However, ICCE and ECCE/IOL may be performed at low cost using simple techniques and appropriate technology. (See Chapter 3 for discussion of locally made surgical lighting, instrumentation, and expendable supplies. Refer to the end of this chapter for a list of essential instrumentation and supplies for cataract surgery.)

Ophthalmologists usually perform most cataract operations. In many African nations, however, clinical officers, medical assistants, and nurses have been trained to perform various kinds of intraocular surgery including cataract surgery. This strategy greatly extends ophthalmic surgical staffing in a region where there is only one ophthalmologist for approximately 1 million people. (See Chapter 1 for discussion of selection of appropriate candidates for surgical training; see Appendix C for basic surgical guidelines for use by ophthalmic medical auxiliaries so trained.)

Optical power of the extracted cataract may be replaced with the following:

- Spectacles. For patients who have undergone bilateral cataract extraction, this is the most practical and economical method of correcting vision.
- Contact lenses. In special circumstances, a contact lens fitted properly on the cornea can correct the refractive error after cataract extraction.
- Intraocular lenses (IOLs). Excellent correction of visual acuity after cataract surgery can be achieved by the implantation of an artificial lens in the eye at the time of cataract surgery.

Indications for cataract surgery

All patients who are blind or visually disabled from cataract are candidates for surgery. A reasonable guideline is to perform cataract extraction on any patient who is unable to carry out normal daily activities because of impaired vision due to cataract.

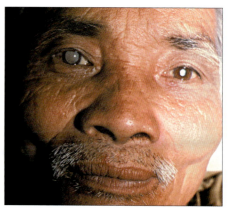

46 Bilateral mature cataract patient, Vietnam.

The specific indications are as follows:

- In most circumstances, if IOL implantation is unavailable, a patient with one normally sighted eye and an immature cataract in the opposite eye with visual impairment is not a candidate for ICCE.
- If visual demands for work (such as driving a motor vehicle) are great, an IOL may be implanted in a monocular aphake.
- If the examiner cannot obtain a good red reflex with the ophthalmoscope and cannot examine the ocular fundus because of media opacity, it is unlikely that the patient has functional vision. If the media opacity is due to cataract, then cataract extraction is indicated.
- All intumescent, hypermature, and Morgagnian cataracts should be extracted (**46**). These advanced cataracts can leak lens protein through the capsule, which can cause secondary phacotoxic uveitis and glaucoma.
- A secondary traumatic cataract should be removed if it causes intraocular complications.
- Advanced bilateral congenital cataracts should be operated on early in life.
- *Aniseikonia* is a difference in the size of the visual image in the two eyes, causing the inability to see a single image with both eyes. This may occur after ICCE in one eye only with aphakic spectacle correction. Aniseikonia is confusing and annoying to the patient. An IOL or a contact lens for aphakic correction in one eye can eliminate aniseikonia in the aphakic patient.

General surgical technique

Although cataract surgery is a rather simple operation, it must be performed very gently and with great care. The eye is a small and delicate organ, and it can easily be permanently damaged by careless surgery. The surgeon must be attentive at all times to all surgical maneuvers to help avoid intraocular complications and must always watch the operating field when holding surgical instruments near or in the eye. *Never move the hand quickly or suddenly in or near the surgical field*.

The surgical assistant should be thoroughly familiar with the operative procedure and with the particular surgeon's technique and preferences. The assistant must anticipate the operation step by step and hand the correct instruments to the surgeon.

If only a limited number of surgical gloves are available, gloves may be worn for several procedures but the hands and gloves must be rinsed in antiseptic solution before every operation. If surgical gloves are not available, the surgeon and assistant may operate bare-handed but must observe strict sterile technique. In bare-handed technique, fingernails should be cut short and be absolutely clean. *Strict surgical scrubbing should be observed*. Hands should also be rinsed after scrubbing with antiseptic solution (methyl alcohol or iodine-based surgical solution).

Tips of fingers should never touch the eye or the ocular adnexa after surgical preparation or during the operation. Fingers – even gloved – should never touch the tips of instruments that will be touching or entering the eye.

When injecting air or sterile solution into the anterior chamber, be certain that the cannula is free of small particles and that the solution is fresh. *First push air or fluid in the syringe through the cannula outside the sterile field before inserting it into the anterior chamber.* This will remove debris from the cannula and can prevent intraocular contamination and possible infection.

Preoperative considerations

Preoperative care

Laboratory studies for preoperative medical evaluation should be selective and performed only for specific complaints or suspected illnesses. Routine screening investigations are expensive and often do not contribute to proper patient care. Measurement of vital signs is a requirement. Systemic blood pressure and pulse rate should be measured. Abnormal blood pressure should be controlled prior to any elective intraocular operation because of the risk of systemic cardiovascular complications intraoperatively. Systemic illness and all infections should be controlled before elective intraocular surgery is undertaken.

A complete ocular examination is necessary before cataract surgery. Be especially aware of the possibility of glaucoma in older patients with cataract. Coexisting disease such as glaucoma and diabetes mellitus can significantly complicate cataract surgery.

Preoperative ocular care (modified appropriately for in-hospital or same-day surgery) includes the following:

- Mydriatic drops (tropicamide, cyclopentolate, phenylephrine, or homatropine) are applied to the eye to be operated on to dilate the pupil.
- Antibiotic drops or ointment (tetracycline ointment or chloramphenicol drops) are applied every 12 hours to both eyes.
- The patient's face should be washed daily with soap and clean water.
- IOP-lowering agents (oral acetazolamide and timolol maleate drops) should be administered if IOP is elevated. Pilocarpine should not be given prior to cataract surgery because the miosis (pupillary constriction) makes cataract surgery difficult.

Pilocarpine also causes vascular congestion, which can cause undue microvascular bleeding during surgery.
- If the eye has been treated for elevated IOP preoperatively, IOP measurement with a sterile Schiøtz tonometer should be performed (see Chapter 16). The IOP should be within the normal range (10–21 mmHg) before entering the eye. If the IOP is over 21 mmHg, the need for surgery should be re-evaluated. *Gentle* external ocular finger massage for 1 minute with the eyelids closed may be able to lower the IOP. A pressure cuff secured by an expandable strap or a balanced counterweight may also be used. An eye with IOP that cannot be lowered should undergo intraocular surgery only in an emergency (such as phacotoxic ocular hypertension).
- Written permission for surgery (informed consent) should be obtained from the patient. The patient and the patient's family should be counseled about the surgery and care of the eyes after surgery.

For efficiency, the patient, if able, may walk to the operating table with assistance.

Anesthesia and akinesia

Paralysis of the eyelids and ocular adnexa and local anesthesia are required for intraocular surgery. General anesthesia is almost never required for adult patients and should be reserved for uncooperative adults with ocular emergencies and for children. Adults may be lightly premedicated with 5 mg of diazepam given orally. The patient should not be medicated to the point of causing sleep.

External and ocular anesthesia and akinesia are achieved as follows:

- Apply one drop of topical anesthetic to the cornea.
- Mix 20 cc lidocaine hydrochloride 1 or 2% with one drop of 1:10,000 epinephrine (adrenaline). Epinephrine delays absorption of the anesthetic.
- For peribulbar block, inject a total of 2–3 cc of this solution in one or more orbital quadrants. Avoid using excessive volume in retrobulbar anesthesia; too much solution in the space behind the eye will push the eyeball forward and will cause undue positive pressure when the eye is opened and possibly contribute to operative complications.
- Inject the eyelids at the orbital rims with 2–3 cc of this solution. If 0.25 cc of hyaluronidase is added to the lidocaine/epinephrine solution, eyelid block may not be necessary. (Hyaluronidase spreads the action of the local block; hence, local anesthetic with hyaluronidase when injected in the peribulbar space usually diffuses sufficiently to also block eyelid movement.)

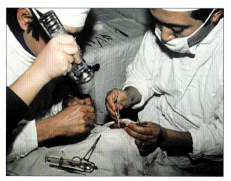

47 Intracapsular cataract extraction at a rural hospital in Vietnam; gloves were not available; the surgeons observe strict sterile technique and never touch the tips of the instruments or the adnexae with their fingers.

- If the eye is congested, apply one drop of topical epinephrine 1:10,000 to the conjunctiva for vasoconstriction of conjunctival vessels. *If the patient is hypertensive, avoid this, because topical epinephrine can cause a sudden rise in blood pressure, which may be followed by cardiovascular complications.*

Sterility

Sterility of the operating field must be maintained with the following steps:

1 The surgeon and assistant must do a thorough 10-minute hand and forearm surgical scrub. Surgical gowns should be worn if available. Whether or not gloves are used, the surgeon and assistant must observe strict 'no touch' surgical technique, taking particular care not to touch the operating field or the tips of surgical instruments (**47**).
2 The face and head of the patient are then wiped with surgical disinfectant and draped in a sterile manner with freshly sterilized surgical linen (or sterile disposable drapes if available).
3 The eyelids are retracted with a small mechanical retractor. Place a single 4-0 superior rectus bridle suture and rotate the eyeball downward by retracting the suture and securing it with snap forceps on the drape.
4 The eyelid margins and ocular surface should then be inspected for debris and mucus. If foreign matter is present, it must be removed using a sterile cotton-tipped applicator, sterile gauze, or irrigation with sterile solution.
5 Thoroughly irrigate the external ocular surfaces and both fornices with sterile saline. These last two steps are important for reducing the risk of intraocular infection by removing residual foreign matter and surface bacteria.

Prior to surgically entering the eye

Immediately before surgically opening the eye, do the following:

- Confirm that no retrobulbar hemorrhage has occurred as a result of the peribulbar anesthetic injection. If the eye is bulging forward or if blood has appeared under the conjunctiva, surgery should be postponed until the peribulbar or retrobulbar hemorrhage has cleared.
- Check that the pupil has been adequately dilated by the drops. If the pupil remains reactive to light, instill cycloplegic drops again.

Intraoperative technique

Intracapsular cataract extraction (ICCE) and extracapsular cataract extraction with intraocular lens implantation (ECCE/IOL) are two procedures that are increasingly practical in the developing world. They are described in depth in the sections that follow.

Phacoemulsification, an ECCE technique in which the lens is dissolved by ultrasound and aspirated, is technically more difficult to perform than manual ECCE/IOL. Because of the high cost of instrumentation and backup systems required for phacoemulsification, it is impractical for use in most parts of the world where cataract remains the major cause of blindness. *Table 5* provides a summary comparison of ICCE, ECCE/IOL, and phacoemulsification/IOL.

Table 5 **Comparison between ICCE, ECCE/IOL, and phacoemulsification/IOL**

	ICCE	ECCE/IOL	Phacoemulsification/IOL
Equipment	Simple	More complicated	Most complex
Illumination/magnification	Loupes	Coaxial light microscope	Coaxial light microscope
Skills	+	++	++++
Complexity	+	++	+++
Support system	+	++	++++
Maintenance (of equipment)	+	+	++++
Spectacles required postoperatively	Yes	Often	Often
Immediate postoperative results	Adequate	Best: equivalent to phaco/IOL	Best: equivalent to ECCE/IOL
Results after 6 months	Lesser	Greater	Greater
Complications	+	++	+++
Posterior capsule present	No	Yes	Yes
Follow-up	Advisable	Required	Required
Nd:YAG required	No	Often	Often
Cost, short term	+	++	++++
Cost, long term (aphakic spectacles)	++	+	+

Intracapsular cataract extraction

Intracapsular cataract extraction (ICCE) is an operation to remove a cataractous lens from the eye in its entirety within its capsule (**48**). The lens may be removed by any of the following methods:

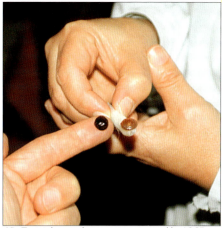

48 Two advanced cataracts extracted by ICCE.

- Cryoextraction is a safe and widely practiced method of extracting a cataractous lens. An ice probe that freezes to the lens capsule provides an attachment to the lens for its removal from the eye. A cryoextraction unit that can be manufactured at low cost is described in Chapter 13.
- Capsule forceps may be used to grasp the anterior surface of the cataract for extraction. Unwanted tearing of the anterior lens capsule, a complication of ICCE, can easily result from forceps delivery.
- An erysiphake, a hand-held instrument that attaches to the lens by suction, is a simple and safe instrument for ICCE.
- A silica gel pellet may be used. The pellet is gripped with forceps and heated briefly over a flame to make it more hygroscopic before placing it on the lens to be extracted.
- ICCE can be performed by manual expression of the lens, using only pressure at the inferior limbus while simultaneously depressing the superior scleral incision lip. This technique, known as the Smith procedure, has been practiced extensively in countries of the Indian subcontinent. No instruments are inserted into the eye in the Smith procedure. This procedure works best with mature or hypermature cataracts in soft eyes.

If the capsule is unintentionally broken in attempting an ICCE, the surgical procedure is converted to an extracapsular extraction. The operation is then known as an 'unplanned ECCE.'

The basic steps to perform an ICCE are as follows (the exact order will vary, based on specific circumstances):

1 Make a 180° conjunctival peritomy (fornix-based flap) from the 9 o'clock to the 3 o'clock position superiorly.
2 Remove the conjunctiva and Tenon's capsule completely from the limbus to a distance of 2.0 mm.
3 Apply cautery to bleeding points.
4 Enter the anterior chamber gently at the limbus with a surgical blade.
5 Extend the incision 165° with right- and left-handed corneoscleral scissors. (A Graefe knife may be used instead of scissors, reducing the number of manual steps from three to one.) A shelved incision may be used or not; refer to ECCE/IOL description below.
6 Perform a single peripheral iridectomy at the 12 o'clock position (to prevent pupillary block, a possible postoperative complication). The iris to be excised is gently elevated at the scleral lip through the corneoscleral incision. It is not necessary to elevate the cornea at the same time.

7 Place a single 9-0 or 10-0 suture through the cornea and sclera at 12 o'clock. A loop from this incision is drawn outside the corneoscleral incision. The assistant gently elevates the cornea by retracting an arm of this suture with forceps.

8 The surgeon dries the remaining aqueous from the anterior chamber with a cellulose sponge and retracts the iris with the sponge. Avoid routine irrigation of the anterior chamber to reduce the risk of intraocular infection. If the anterior chamber must be irrigated to remove lens fragments (if the procedure becomes an unplanned ECCE/IOL) or to reform the anterior chamber, a millipore filter can be used between the syringe and the tip when irrigating. The filter will remove bacteria and contaminated particles from the solution. Millipore filters are expensive and often difficult to obtain. They should be used only once and discarded. Never reuse a millipore filter. Be especially alert to possible bacterial contamination of solutions produced locally by hospital pharmacies. *A contaminated solution used for anterior chamber irrigation can cause postoperative endophthalmitis (intraocular infection) and permanent loss of the eye.*

9 Irrigate 2 ml of alpha-chymotrypsin solution (if available) into the posterior chamber for lysis of the zonules if necessary. Adults younger than 50 years of age often require alpha-chymotrypsin; it is generally not required for those over 50 years of age. Irrigate out the enzyme after 1 minute.

10 Remove the cataract by cryoextraction, or with an erysiphake, capsule forceps, or a silica gel pellet if a cryoextraction unit is not available. Capsule forceps should not be used for intracapsular extraction of hypermature or Morgagnian cataracts because of the risk of tearing the anterior capsule. The Smith procedure (manual expression) may be substituted for hypermature or Morgagnian cataracts. Note the following points :

■ Separate the lens from the zonules by gently applying pressure at the inferior limbus at 6 o'clock with a muscle hook and stripping to 9 o'clock and 3 o'clock as the lens is being delivered.

■ Extreme care must be exercised during the extraction to avoid touching the corneal endothelium. *Damaging the endothelium can cause permanent corneal edema.*

■ If the anterior capsule is inadvertently torn, the procedure is converted to an ECCE (see below). If no IOL is available, leave the posterior capsule in place.

■ If vitreous appears in the anterior chamber or is disturbed, an anterior vitrectomy must be performed. This may be done with one of several different automated cutting and aspirating instruments or with cellulose sponges and scissors.

11 Draw the single 9-0 or 10-0 suture down and tie it and rotate the suture knot to the scleral side of the incision. Place an additional three or four interrupted sutures in the incision, and rotate and bury all suture knots in the sclera to prevent irritation to the eyelids.

12 Any iris trapped in the incision must be repositioned into the anterior chamber using a flat spatula.

13 If the anterior chamber is not formed at the completion of the surgical wound closure, a small amount of air may be injected. Be careful because too much air will elevate the IOP. Avoid reforming the anterior chamber with solution if sterility of the solution is questionable.

14 Inspect the wound closure by gently depressing the sclera with a forceps tip 2.0 mm posterior to the incision at several points. If gentle pressure produces a leak of aqueous, additional sutures are required to seal the leak.

15 Cut one arm of the bridle suture near the superior rectus and then draw the conjunctiva down over the surgical incision. Sutures to repair the conjunctiva can irritate the eyelid margins and are usually not necessary.

16 Instill a mydriatic (atropine 1%, if available) and an antibiotic drop or ointment (tetracycline 1%) in the inferior fornix. Subconjunctival injections of gentamicin and corticosteroid solutions are not used unless indicated by a surgical complication or preexisting ocular condition.

17 Dress the eye with a double sterile pad and a shield produced from discarded X-ray film, heavy paper, or light cardboard (see Chapter 3).

18 Assist the patient in walking from the operating room to the recovery area.

ICCE with anterior chamber IOL implantation

After performing an uncomplicated ICCE, an open-loop anterior chamber IOL may be implanted, as follows:

1 Place several 10-0 sutures in the scleral incision to partially close it, leaving an area of the central incision unsutured for IOL implantation.

2 Deepen the anterior chamber with sterile solution or viscoelastic using a fine cannula on a syringe.

3 Grasp the anterior chamber IOL with nontoothed forceps and inspect it under the microscope for defects such as scratches or jagged edges. If the IOL is suitable for implantation, insert the open-loop IOL into the anterior chamber over a lens glide and position the feet of the inferior haptic in the inferior angle.

4 Remove the lens glide and position the feet of the superior haptic in the superior angle with forceps.

5 'Walk' the IOL 90° (reposition it in small steps using a lens hook) so that the open loops and feet are positioned at the 3 and 9 o'clock positions (horizontal) in the anterior chamber.

6 If viscoelastic has been used, irrigate it from the anterior chamber using a fine cannula on a syringe.

7 Close the scleral incision with 3–4 interrupted 10-0 nylon sutures to achieve a fluid-tight wound (no leakage).

8 Follow through from step 14 on as described above.

Extracapsular cataract extraction with intraocular lens implantation (ECCE/IOL)

In ECCE/IOL the anterior lens capsule is opened and/or removed, the lens cortex and nucleus are removed, and the posterior lens capsule is left in place to support an IOL which is implanted in the posterior chamber. If the posterior lens capsule is torn and cannot support a posterior chamber IOL, an anterior chamber IOL can be implanted.

ECCE /IOL has become a common operation in developing nations. The development of high-quality and reasonably priced IOLs and coaxial light surgical microscopes has made this possible.

The preoperative preparation for ECCE/IOL is the same as for ICCE. The steps to perform ECCE/IOL are as follows (the exact order will depend on circumstances):

1 Make a 180° conjunctival peritomy (fornix-based flap) from the 9 o'clock to the 3 o'clock position superiorly (**49**).
2 Remove conjunctival remnants and Tenon's capsule completely from the limbus to a distance of 2.0 mm.
3 Apply cautery to bleeding points (**50**).
4 Incise the sclera 1.5 mm posterior to the limbus to 0.5 mm in depth and extend this incision to 165°. Dissect forward until clear cornea is reached. Do not enter the eye (**51**).
5 Enter the anterior chamber gently with a corneal knife or keratome to the width of 1.5–2.0 mm (**52**).
6 If the anterior chamber is shallow, it should be deepened with sterile solution or viscoelastic through a fine cannula from a small syringe (**53**). If sterile fluids are not available, air may be used to deepen the chamber (**54**).

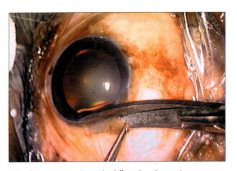

49 Create a conjunctival flap (peritomy).

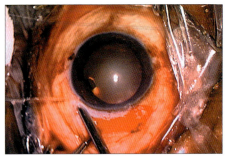

50 Apply a thermal cautery to scleral vessels.

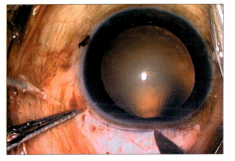

51 Create a grooved incision half the depth of the sclera. Do not enter the anterior chamber.

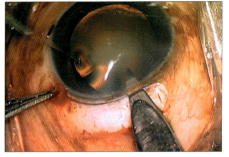

52 Enter the anterior chamber with a keratome or surgical blade.

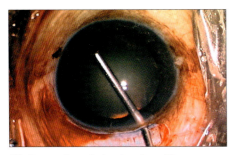

53 Deepen the anterior chamber with viscoelastic.

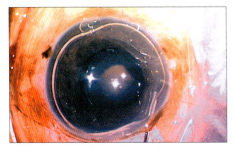

54 Use air if viscoelastic is not available.

7 Using a 30-gauge needle with a bent tip (or a cystotome if available), create an anterior capsulotomy by making a series of puncture marks in the anterior capsule of the lens in a circle of 6.0 mm to 7.0 mm diameter (**55, 56**). Remove the circle of the central anterior capsule with fine forceps.

8 Carry out hydrodissection with sterile saline or balanced salt solution through a fine cannula inserted under the inferior anterior capsule margin to separate the remaining capsule from the cortex and nucleus.

9 Extend the incision with corneoscleral scissors to 165° so that the incision is shelved in its entire length (**57**). A shelved incision allows more scleral tissue to come in contact during the healing process.

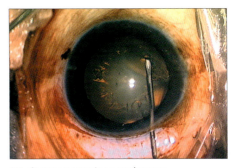

56 Create an anterior capsulotomy.

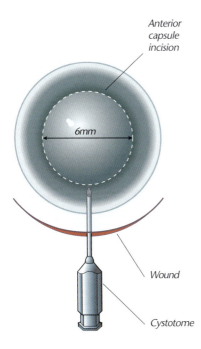

Anterior capsule incision

6mm

Wound

Cystotome

55 Anterior capsulotomy using a cystotome.

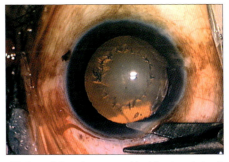

57 Extend the sclero-corneal incision in a shelved fashion.

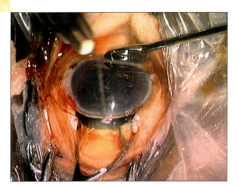

58 Deliver the nucleus with gentle counter-pressure and depression of the scleral lip.

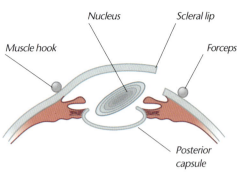

Nucleus   Scleral lip

Muscle hook   Forceps

Posterior capsule

59 Side view of nucleus expression.

10 Draw the superior rectus bridle suture that was placed preoperatively snugly downward and secure it with a mosquito forceps so that the scleral lip at the 12 o'clock position is slightly open.

11 Using light pressure at the 6 o'clock position with a muscle hook and depression of the scleral lip with fine forceps at 12 o'clock, express the nucleus from its position within the crystalline lens through the anterior chamber and out of the eye (58, 59).

Note the following points:

■ This step must be performed gently, without force. Undue pressure can extend the anterior capsulotomy to the posterior capsule, causing a tear in the posterior capsule.
■ Extreme care must be taken to avoid touching or damaging the corneal endothelium. *Damage to the endothelium can cause permanent corneal edema.*

12 Release the bridle suture from its secured position held by mosquito forceps and allow the scleral lip to relax.

13 Irrigate loose cortex from the anterior chamber and the scleral incision with sterile solution.

14 Close the scleral incision by placing, securing, and tying 3–4 interrupted 10-0 sutures to achieve a fluid-tight wound (no leakage).

15 Using a hand-held aspiration/irrigation device, perform aspiration of the lens cortex (60). Again, great care must be taken with this step. All movements inside the eye must be carried out carefully and with precision. Every attempt must be made to preserve the posterior capsule intact and to remove only cortex from the capsular bag. If capsular tissue is inadvertently sucked into the aspiration tip port, stop the aspiration temporarily (the tissue must be irrigated and not pulled out of the eye with the instrument).

16 After all cortex is removed from the capsular bag and the anterior chamber, deepen the anterior chamber and the capsular bag with sterile solution or viscoelastic.

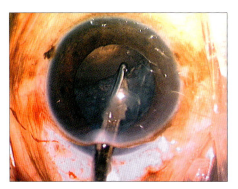

60 Aspiration of cortical material.

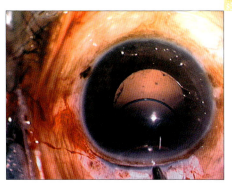

61 Implant the intraocular lens into the capsular bag.

17 Remove the suture at the 12 o'clock position at the scleral incision.

18 Grasp the posterior chamber IOL with nontoothed forceps and inspect it under the microscope for defects such as scratches or uneven edges. If the IOL is suitable for implantation, slip it through the scleral incision and position the inferior haptic in the capsular bag (**61, 62**).

19 Grasp the superior haptic near its free end with a smooth forceps, introduce it into the anterior chamber, position it behind the superior iris, and release it (**63**) .

20 Using a fine cannula on a syringe, irrigate the anterior chamber with sterile solution, removing all visco-elastic and cortical remnants from the anterior chamber (**64**).

21 If capsular remnants remain in the anterior chamber, they should not be pulled out, but instead excised with fine intraocular scissors and removed gently. Pulling on an anterior capsular remnant can extend and tear the posterior capsule.

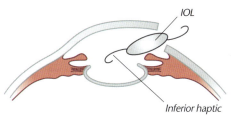

62 Side view of IOL implantation.

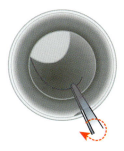

63 Grasp the superior haptic with smooth forceps and depress it posterior to the iris before releasing.

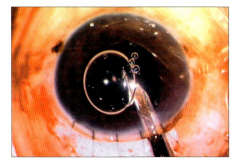

64 Irrigate the anterior chamber with sterile solution to remove any debris.

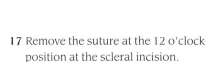

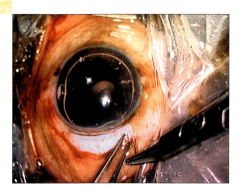

65 Repair the shelved surgical incision.

22 Repair the corneoscleral incision with the interrupted 10-0 sutures (**65**). The sutures should be placed 1.5 mm posterior to the wound edges and half the depth of the sclera. All knots should be rotated and buried in the sclera to prevent irritation to the eyelids.

23 Inspect the wound closure by gently depressing the sclera with a forceps tip 2 mm posterior to the incision at several points. If aqueous fluid leaks from the wound with gentle pressure, additional sutures are required to close the scleral incision.

24 Remove the bridle suture by cutting near the loop under the superior rectus muscle so as not to draw the remaining suture under the muscle.

25 Apply topical dexamethasone 1% and tetracycline 1% ointment to the inferior fornix.

26 Dress the eye with a double sterile pad and a shield produced from discarded x-ray film, heavy paper, or light cardboard (see Chapter 3).

27 Allow the patient to walk with assistance from the operating room to the recovery area.

Intraoperative complications of ICCE and ECCE/IOL

The following complications occur intraoperatively; there is overlap between these and complications that occur postoperatively (next section):

- *Dialysis of the iris root.* The iris may separate from its attachment to the sclera or be inadvertently incised with a surgical knife or scissors when making the corneal entrance incision. This may result in a difficult surgery or impaired vision if the iris drops over the visual axis postoperatively. The anterior chamber must be kept deep and the surgeon must carefully watch the tips of all instruments within the eye to avoid this complication.

- *Hyphema.* Persistent bleeding from vessels in the scleral wound may cause intraoperative hyphema, obscuring the surgeon's view and ability to operate. Cauterize the bleeding scleral vessels and carefully lavage the free blood from the anterior chamber. Do not pull out blood clots that are attached to the iris, because the iris may be torn if the clots are attached firmly while an attempt is made to remove them.

- *Flat anterior chamber.* A shallow or flat anterior chamber makes surgery difficult. It is usually due to high IOP or pressure on the globe from pressure from the eyelids. Loosen the bridle suture and elevate the eyelid speculum to lessen the IOP. Inject sterile solution or viscoelastic to deepen the anterior chamber. A shallow or flat anterior chamber may be prevented by extending the eyelid fissure temporally with a preoperative incision at the lateral canthus (lateral canthotomy).

- *Corneal endothelial damage.* Corneal opacity from edema can be avoided if the endothelium is protected during surgery. Operating in a deep and well-formed anterior chamber can help prevent endothelial damage. Exercise extreme care to avoid touching the corneal endothelium during cataract surgery.
- *Posterior capsule tear.* A complication of planned ECCE/IOL only, a tear in the posterior capsule during ECCE/IOL often requires vitrectomy to remove vitreous that bulges forward into the anterior chamber. After anterior vitrectomy, a posterior chamber IOL may be implanted in front of the anterior lens capsule or an anterior chamber IOL may be used instead.

Postoperative considerations

Postoperative care should be directed toward maintaining a clean and healthy postoperative eye. Healing and visual rehabilitation usually require 4–5 weeks. For ICCE patients, if the surgical patient lives a great distance from the hospital and is unlikely to return for follow-up, refraction and fitting with aphakic (high convex, or 'plus') spectacles may be done at the time of hospital discharge. If an ECCE patient can return 1 month after surgery, refraction may be performed at that time and spectacles given to correct the residual refractive error.

Routine care and findings

On the first postoperative day, the cornea may be slightly cloudy and the conjunctiva congested. The anterior chamber should be deep.

Pain on the first postoperative day may indicate high intraocular pressure. If the eye is painful, tonometry must be performed. If the IOP is elevated, treat with acetazolamide and topical timolol maleate until IOP returns to normal.

The cornea and conjunctiva should clear rapidly. If pain and chemosis (edema of the conjunctiva) are present and are worse on the second and third days after surgery, an eye-threatening infection (endophthalmitis) may be present and must be managed immediately.

The postoperative cataract patient should be encouraged to walk and exercise on the first postoperative day and daily while in the hospital. The dressing should be changed at the time of examination on the first postoperative day. A sturdy shield with one or more pinholes may be used to protect the operated eye at night while the patient is sleeping and during the day for 3 weeks thereafter if the patient desires (see Chapter 3). The patient must be told not to rub or touch the operated eye.

In uncomplicated cataract surgery, atropine 1% ointment and tetracycline 1% ointment are instilled once daily, and topical corticosteroids are instilled two or three times daily for postoperative inflammation for 2 weeks or for the length of time the patient is in hospital. Subconjunctival corticosteroids are used immediately postoperatively especially if vitreous has been lost. Do not give the patient ocular corticosteroids for outpatient use after cataract surgery unless postoperative inflammation is still present when the patient is discharged from the hospital.

Complications of ICCE

A variety of postoperative complications may occur after an uncomplicated cataract operation. Daily examination of the operated eye is necessary to diagnose these complications. Although serious postoperative complications are not common, the ophthalmic practitioner must be able to recognize and treat them:

- *Hyphema.* Blood in the anterior chamber (see Figure 99, page 133) may be present on the first postoperative day or soon after. Treat with continued antibiotic and atropine treatment and patching of both eyes with pads to put the eyes at rest. The patient should be confined to bed when bilaterally patched.
- *Iritis.* Postoperative iritis is recognized by ciliary flush (vascular injection at the limbus) and pain. Cells and flare are seen in the anterior chamber with the slit lamp. Continue atropine treatment. Treat with topical corticosteroids if the inflammation is mild or subconjunctival corticosteroids if the inflammation is severe.
- *Elevated IOP.* IOP can rise after an uncomplicated cataract extraction. It is important to establish the cause of the IOP elevation.

  If the IOP elevation is secondary to alpha-chymotrypsin used during surgery, the IOP will return to normal in a few days. Timolol maleate or acetazolamide can be used to lower the IOP until the effect of the alpha-chymotrypsin diminishes.

  Pupillary block can occur if the peripheral iridectomy is blocked. The iris and vitreous are pushed forward and the anterior chamber is shallow. Full dilation of the pupil with mydriatics may break the attack. If this does not work, surgery is necessary to break pupillary block.

- *Iris prolapse.* Prolapse of iris through the corneoscleral section can occur, especially if the patient touches or rubs the eye in the early postoperative period. The prolapsed iris should be repositioned immediately under sterile conditions in the operating room.
- *Shallow anterior chamber.* A shallow anterior chamber in the immediate postoperative period may be caused by any of the following:

1 Wound leak. To diagnose this complication, place a small quantity of fluorescein on the superior limbus and gently press the eyeball on the inferior eyelid with a cotton-tipped applicator (Seidel test). Leaking aqueous will be visible in the fluorescein pattern. The IOP usually will be low (less than 10 mmHg). If the anterior chamber is shallow or flat, surgical repair of the wound leak is required.

2 Pupillary block. With pupillary block, the IOP is high, the anterior chamber is shallow or flat, and there is no wound leak (the wound leak test is negative). A peripheral iridectomy may be necessary.

3 Choroidal effusion. Fluid between the choroid and sclera postoperatively will cause bulging or ballooning in the periphery of the red reflex, visible with the direct ophthalmoscope. Surgical drainage of this fluid may be necessary if the choroidal effusion is not reduced in size in 5 days.

- *Endophthalmitis.* Salvaging an eye with endophthalmitis will usually depend on early diagnosis, identification of the bacterium, and correct therapy. Clinical signs of endophthalmitis usually appear on the second or third postoperative day. Swelling of the conjunctiva (chemosis) and pain are early signs. Heavy cells and flare are visible with the slit lamp, and hypopyon (pus cells layered in the inferior anterior chamber) is evident. Purulent discharge (pus) may be present on the ocular surface.

  Identify the bacterium if possible. Culture conjunctival discharge on a bacteriologic culture plate. Also culture the aqueous. Anterior chamber fluid may be obtained by paracentesis (aspirating a small amount of aqueous through the limbus) with a 27-gauge needle on a syringe. The aspirate should be cultured and a Gram's stain performed. A vitreous tap through the pars plana should also be taken and cultured. A Gram's stain should also be performed on the vitreous aspirate. Treat the bacterial infection according to the results of the Gram's stain and culture and bacterial sensitivities. (See Chapter 11 for directions on obtaining a Gram's stain.)

  Do not wait for laboratory results. Begin treatment immediately with daily subconjunctival injections of gentamicin 1.0 cc and dexamethasone 1.0 cc (to reduce inflammation and contraction of the vitreous), and topical chloramphenicol drops hourly. Atropine 1% should be administered topically every 12 hours.

  Vitrectomy through the sclera can sometimes be performed at tertiary hospital centers. In most rural surgical services, vitrectomy equipment is not available.

- *Retinal detachment.* Retinal detachment occurs infrequently as a complication of cataract surgery. Showers of 'sparks,' a 'curtain,' and clouded vision with decreased visual acuity (if the detachment includes the macula) are symptoms. Pain is not a symptom. Early diagnosis and surgical reattachment of the retina are necessary to restore and preserve vision.

- *Cystoid macular edema (CME).* CME presents as a raised macular area with decreased visual acuity. It may accompany disturbance of the vitreous after ECCE/IOL but also occurs more frequently after ICCE. Treat CME with topical corticosteroids and anti-inflammatory drugs.

Complications of ECCE/IOL

These comments are supplementary to the discussion of ICCE complications, especially as related to the use of intraocular lenses:

- *Hyphema.* Blood in the anterior chamber may follow ECCE/IOL. It may originate from vessels in the scleral wound or from a vessel tear in the iris. Place the patient on bed rest with a full-time occlusive patch until the hyphema clears.
- *Uveitis.* Anterior uveitis is a common complication of ECCE/IOL. Use a cycloplegic drop twice a day and a topical corticosteroid drop at least four times a day until cells and flare in the anterior chamber clear. Corticosteroid drops may be used more frequently if the uveitis is severe.
- *Wound leak.* Hypotony (IOP less than 10 mmHg) usually indicates a wound leak. Check the wound for a leak with gentle pressure at the wound edge using a cotton-tipped applicator and sterile fluorescein dye (Seidel test). Patching for 2–3 days may hasten wound closure and healing. If hypotony persists, additional sutures in the wound may be necessary to achieve closure and to stop the leak.
- *Corneal edema.* Corneal edema lasting several days is a frequent occurrence after ECCE/IOL and may be related to elevated IOP. If so, treat the ocular hypertension with topical antihypertensive drops (do not use miotics) and acetazolamide tablets. Persistent corneal edema may result from damage to the corneal endothelium. An eye with a permanently cloudy cornea following IOL surgery may require a corneal transplant.

- *Retained lens matter.* If the posterior capsule has been torn during surgery, cortex or nuclear fragments may be retained in the vitreous. If the posterior capsule is intact, lens remnants, usually cortex, may be retained in the anterior chamber, and secondary anterior uveitis may result. Treat with topical mydriatics and corticosteroids until the cortical material has absorbed.
- *Elevated IOP.* If viscoelastic has been used and has not been completely irrigated out of the anterior chamber after ECCE/IOL, IOP may be elevated postoperatively. It usually lasts only a few days. If the IOP remains high, treat with topical antihypertensives (but not miotics) and acetazolamide. In addition, capsular and cortical remnants from ECCE may block the trabecular meshwork and elevate the IOP. Treat with topical corticosteroids, atropine, and timolol maleate. Acetazolamide may be added for additional IOP control.
- *Pupillary capture.* The iris may tuck behind the posterior chamber IOL if the IOL tilts forward when the pupil is dilated. The pupil will be distorted (not round). If there is no inflammation, IOP is normal, and the iris is not pulled over the center of the IOL, there is no reason to surgically reposition the IOL.
- *Cystoid macular edema (CME).* Although CME may follow ECCE/IOL, it occurs more frequently after ICCE. It presents as a raised macular area with decreased visual acuity. Treat with topical anti-inflammatory drops. Cystoid macular edema may clear spontaneously in several weeks without treatment.
- *Posterior capsule opacification.* Clouding of the posterior lens capsule that supports the posterior chamber

IOL frequently occurs months to years after IOL implantation, causing clouding of vision. If the clouding of vision is significant, the capsule should be opened. This may be performed with an Nd:YAG laser. Alternatively, a cystotome (a thin wire probe with a hooked, pointed tip) may be passed into the anterior vitreous space through the pars plana to incise or open the cloudy capsule to clear the visual axis. The pars plana capsulotomy should be done under sterile surgical conditions.

- *Retinal detachment.* Separation or detachment of the retina does not occur as frequently after ECCE/IOL as after ICCE.
- *Endophthalmitis.* Endophthalmitis must be diagnosed and treated immediately to save the eye (see under Complications of ICCE).
- *Decentered posterior chamber IOL.* The posterior chamber IOL may be found postsurgically to be off-center. This may be due to a tear in the posterior capsule which allows the IOL to shift position. If the decentered IOL does not create a serious visual disturbance for the patient, it is best not to attempt to surgically recenter it. If it causes monocular diplopia (double vision in one eye only), surgery may again be undertaken to center the IOL or to remove it and replace the posterior chamber IOL with an anterior chamber IOL. This should be undertaken only by an experienced surgeon because of the difficulty of the operation.
- *Dislocated posterior chamber IOL.* An IOL that drops out of a torn capsular bag into the vitreous body should be removed by a surgeon experienced in vitreoretinal surgery. An anterior chamber IOL may then be implanted after vitrectomy is performed.

Surgical equipment

A basic surgical instrumentation and sterilizing kit and a list of expendable supplies for performing intraocular surgery is listed in Appendix D. Many of the supplies and instruments described can be manufactured locally at low cost. See Chapter 3 for details on such techniques.

An operating microscope may be used if available, but good operating loupes provide adequate magnification for ICCE. Operating loupes conserve operating time, are convenient for field work, are inexpensive, and require far less maintenance than an operating microscope. ECCE/IOL requires a coaxial light microscope.

If a formal operating room is not available, any clean room and a body-length table will suffice. A clean water source is necessary.

A high-intensity operating light is also necessary. A halogen motor vehicle headlight may be attached to an intravenous infusion pole and powered by a 12-volt battery for excellent operating illumination in rural settings where electrical power is erratic or unavailable (see Figures 14 and 15 in Chapter 3).

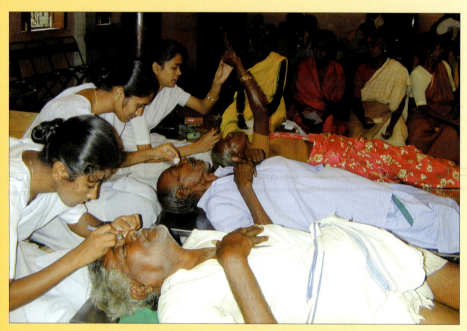

Preoperative Schiøtz tonometry by technicians at Aravind Hospital, India.
Tonometry measures intraocular pressure by determining the resistance of the cornea to indentation: high pressure indicates an increased risk of glaucoma.

6

Glaucoma

Maiyeu na Madooku (I don't want to be a blind man)
East African Masai song

Glaucoma is the second leading cause of blindness in the world. Blindness and low vision resulting from glaucoma can be prevented or delayed by early detection and proper management. A basic knowledge of how glaucoma causes blindness and low vision is necessary to diagnose and manage the various forms of the disease. Awareness of the possibility of the disease, and the suspicion that it might be present, as well as simple but detailed examination techniques, can help in diagnosing glaucoma, treating it appropriately, and preventing blindness.

Introduction, background, and epidemiology

Glaucoma occurs when the intraocular pressure (IOP) exceeds the ability of the affected eye to tolerate it. There is no specific level of IOP that defines glaucoma. In general, the higher the IOP, the greater is the risk of glaucoma and loss of peripheral vision, low vision, and blindness. Damage to the optic nerve (the optic disc) and nerve fibers of the retina results in visual loss. Although the rates of occurrence of glaucoma increase with age, glaucoma may occur at any age. The eye health care worker should always be aware of this potentially blinding disease even in a patient with normal central acuity and a normal external ocular examination.

Because glaucoma may rarely be present at birth (childhood or infantile glaucoma) and may develop at any time during life, glaucoma is known as a 'cradle to the grave' disease. Most forms of glaucoma, however, are more common and increase in prevalence with increasing age.

Glaucoma is worldwide in distribution. The World Health Organization in 2002 calculated that glaucoma was responsible for approximately 12% of blindness worldwide, making it the second leading cause. Approximately 75% of all glaucoma occurs in the developing world. Glaucoma is particularly difficult to diagnose and treat because most low vision and blindness from glaucoma develop slowly and without symptoms. Because of its chronic and silent progression, glaucoma is known as the 'sneak thief of sight.' Open-angle glaucoma is more prevalent and severe in Africa and in peoples of African descent. Angle-closure glaucoma occurs in all racial groups and in all populations, but it is more prevalent in Asians, particularly in China and SE Asia. Although dramatic and painful in its onset, acute angle-closure glaucoma is less common than open-angle glaucoma or chronic angle-closure glaucoma.

Loss of peripheral vision and central acuity from glaucoma, if long standing, is almost always irreversible. Only rarely can lowering intraocular pressure by medical therapy or surgical operation restore vision that has been lost from glaucoma when damage to the optic nerve and nerve fiber layer has occurred.

Visual loss usually occurs in the peripheral visual field and progresses to the central visual field if the disease is not controlled by controlling intraocular pressure. A patient with glaucoma may have good central vision but restricted peripheral vision. Many people with glaucoma are unaware that they are losing vision from glaucoma because their central vision usually remains unchanged from glaucoma until late in the disease process. Symptoms early in chronic glaucoma are usually absent. In acute angle-closure glaucoma symptoms can be dramatic. Screening programs for glaucoma frequently produce false positives and miss the disease when only intraocular pressures are measured.

The 'normal' IOP range is 10–21 mmHg. This is considered normal because the IOP of 95% of eyes measures within this range. Glaucoma may occasionally occur in an eye with IOP within the normal range. This is known as 'low pressure,' 'low tension,' or 'normotensive' glaucoma.

An IOP above 21 mmHg does not necessarily mean that glaucoma is present, but it should be suspected. Until glaucoma is proven, such a patient is considered to be a 'glaucoma suspect,' and if intraocular pressure is above 21 mmHg, then the term 'ocular hypertensive' is used.

These are the major criteria used to establish a diagnosis of glaucoma:

- Elevated IOP (ocular hypertension).
- Characteristic visual field loss.
- Characteristic damage to the optic disc (nerve head) including abnormal cupping and notching (**66**, **67**).

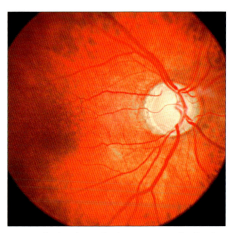

66 Ocular fundus with glaucomatous disc (optic nerve) atrophy.

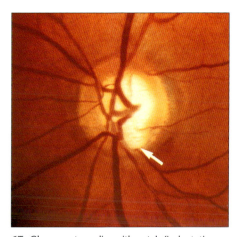

67 Glaucomatous disc with notch (indentation; see arrow) in cup, resulting in loss of peripheral visual field.

Classification

Glaucoma may occur at any age as a 'primary' eye disease. 'Secondary' glaucoma is due to other causes, including trauma, a major cause of unilateral glaucoma. The 'primary' glaucomas – open-angle glaucoma, angle-closure glaucoma (both acute and chronic), and childhood glaucoma – are usually bilateral but may occur unilaterally. An attack of acute angle-closure glaucoma may occur in only one eye, but the potential for an attack in the other eye is great. The following classification is based on clinical findings, age of the patient, and associated or causative disease processes.

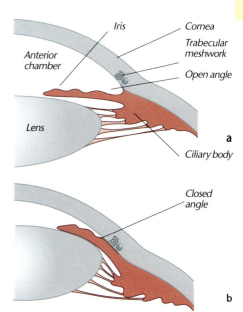

68 Comparison of a) open- angle glaucoma and b) closed-angle glaucoma, where the trabecular meshwork is blocked by the iris and aqueous fluid cannot drain. See also Figure 165.

Primary open-angle glaucoma
Primary open-angle glaucoma is the most common form of glaucoma. The characteristics are as follows:

- The anterior chamber is deep and the drainage angle is open.
- It usually develops in older people. With age, the trabecular meshwork becomes less able to drain aqueous from the anterior chamber (**68a**). When drainage of aqueous is reduced, IOP increases.
- Primary open-angle glaucoma may be inherited.
- It is almost always bilateral but often asymmetric.
- Good central vision is usually preserved until late in the disease, but eventually central vision can also be lost.
- Because the disease is painless and the only symptom early in its course is loss of peripheral vision, patients often do not seek medical attention until late in the disease after vision has already been permanently lost.
- The disease is more prevalent and more severe in patients of African origin or descent.

Angle-closure glaucoma
Angle-closure glaucoma may be chronic (long-standing with few symptoms) or acute (with sudden pain and loss of vision with an acute attack). The characteristics of *chronic* angle-closure glaucoma are as follows:

- Intraocular pressure may be only minimally elevated.
- Visual symptoms (halos and decreased visual acuity) may be only intermittently experienced.
- Severe pain usually is not a feature.
- Results when the trabecular meshwork and drainage angle are partially blocked by iris; peripheral anterior synechiae usually form (**68b**).
- Bilateral.
- Worldwide distribution.
- Most common in Asian populations, particularly in India and China.

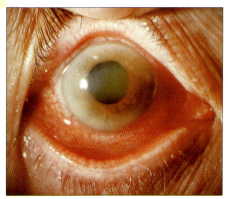

69 Acute angle-closure glaucoma. Note central corneal edema resulting from sudden high intraocular pressure.

The characteristics of *acute* angle-closure glaucoma are as follows:

- Sudden onset.
- Pain and loss of vision are hallmarks.
- Normal iris occludes the trabecular meshwork completely, blocking outflow of aqueous (**68b**).
- High intraocular pressure (**69**).
- Occurs in an eye with an abnormally shallow anterior chamber (see page 105).
- Usually attacks are unilateral but may be bilateral; potential exists in fellow eye for acute attack.
- Worldwide distribution.
- Uncommon in Africans and persons of African descent; more common in Asians and Caucasians.

Secondary glaucoma

Secondary glaucoma includes a variety of glaucomas that result from other causes such as the following:

- Trauma, including penetrating injuries and blunt trauma to the globe, contusion, partially or completely dislocated lens.
- Complications from intraocular surgery, especially cataract surgery.
- Uveitis.
- Neovascularization (growth of abnormal blood vessels) of the iris and angle (from diabetes mellitus, for example).
- Intraocular tumors (rare, but can be responsible for secondary glaucoma).
- Pseudoexfoliation glaucoma (associated with flaking of the lens capsule); occurs frequently in ethnic populations in Africa and the Indian subcontinent.

Childhood glaucoma

Childhood glaucoma (sometimes called 'infantile glaucoma') is present at birth or soon thereafter. The characteristics are as follows:

- Drainage of aqueous from the anterior chamber is blocked by abnormal tissue.
- Infantile glaucoma is nearly always bilateral.
- Infantile glaucoma is rare, but a worldwide problem. It requires early surgical treatment.

Examination, history-taking, and diagnosis

Glaucoma should be suspected in any eye with unexplained visual loss. The diagnosis of glaucoma is often missed or neglected, but awareness of the disease and a detailed ocular examination will identify most cases. Tonometry and examination of the anterior segment structures, the pupils (for afferent pupillary defect), the lens, and the optic nerve are all very important in establishing the diagnosis.

Sophisticated ocular diagnostic tests may not be available. Most patients with glaucoma can be diagnosed by taking a good history and doing a complete ocular examination that includes accurate tonometry. Simple instruments are adequate: a good flashlight (torch); loupe magnification; a direct ophthalmoscope; and a Schiøtz tonometer. If perimetry is not available, an approximate visual field should be obtained (see 'Performing cross-confrontation visual-field testing' below).

The examination begins when the patient enters the examination room. Does the patient require assistance to move about the room? Does the patient use her/his hands to assist in identifying landmarks? Does the patient appear to fix on images and visual targets and hold fixation? Are there blind family members? Has any family member ever been treated for glaucoma? Ask if a family member has been placed on eye drops to control pressure if the term 'glaucoma' is not understood. Other risk factors, in addition to positive family history, include diabetes mellitus (the rate of occurrence of open angle glaucoma is higher in diabetics), people of African descent, and ocular injury.

The pupil size can help in diagnosis. If the pupils are round, regular, and equal in diameter, they should react normally to light stimulus. If the pupil in the affected eye is slow to react to light stimulus, disease in the posterior segment, commonly glaucoma, should be suspected. If the pupil in the affected eye does not constrict when focal light is directed into it after removing the light stimulus from the opposite eye and pupil (and, especially, if the pupil in the affected eye dilates instead of constricts), then glaucoma or posterior segment disease should be suspected. This is the 'afferent pupillary defect,' or 'swinging flashlight' test (and sign). This is an important clinical sign and the test should be performed whenever glaucoma and/or posterior segment disease is suspected.

Primary open-angle glaucoma
History
Often the patient with primary open-angle glaucoma does not seek treatment until late in the course of the disease. Complaints can include loss of peripheral visual field, 'darkness,' halos or rings around lights and redness. Pain may be minimal until late in the disease, at which time IOP becomes markedly elevated and pain may become severe. Long-term topical and systemic use of corticosteroids can cause glaucoma. The family history is important. The presence of glaucoma in first-degree family members (parents, siblings, and descendants) increases the possibility of glaucoma.

Visual acuity
Refraction is necessary if visual loss is in part due to refractive error. Primary open-angle glaucoma tends to be more severe and more rapidly progressive in myopes, particularly high myopes (more than 6 diopters of myopia).

Visual fields
Visual fields can be constricted or reduced. Although it is usually not possible to

perform a detailed visual field examination in a rural eye clinic, an approximate measurement of visual fields is important for diagnosis (see 'Performing cross-confrontation visual-field testing' below).

Observation

Patients with advanced glaucoma will often have difficulty walking without assistance. This is because visual acuity is likely reduced and the visual field is greatly constricted. This can be in contrast with a patient with cataracts who has poor vision but is still able to walk without assistance because of a full visual field. Direct observation of how a patient is able to walk unassisted can be made when the patient enters the examination room. Did the patient require an assistant to walk and to find the way? Did the patient extend his/her hands to guide about furniture or obstacles? Did the patient move the head in a searching motion to better visualize objects in their path? Was it more difficult for the patient to walk in low illumination?

Microscopic examination of the anterior segment

Slit-lamp examination should be performed to diagnose other intraocular disease; loupe magnification may be used if a slit lamp is not available. Cataract is commonly associated with glaucoma because both glaucoma and cataract tend to occur in older age groups. Secondary glaucoma should be suspected if there is evidence of injury and/or intraocular inflammation. Flaking of the anterior lens capsule may indicate pseudoexfoliation. Blood vessels in the iris may indicate neovascularization. The depth of the anterior chamber should be noted with the slit lamp beam. The pupillary size and reaction should be noted. Does the patient have an afferent pupil? (The 'swinging flashlight sign'; see page 103 and Glossary.)

Tonometry

Several techniques are available including the applanation method with the slit lamp or with various hand-held instruments. The simplest and most widely available tonometer in the developing world is the Schiøtz indentation tonometer (its use is described in detail in Chapter 16). The tonopen is a convenient portable tonometer.

Gonioscopy

This is a method of examination of the drainage angle and trabecular meshwork with a special lens placed on the corneal surface. A slit lamp and other special instruments are necessary for this examination. If the angle is not visible, angle-closure glaucoma must be suspected.

Ophthalmoscopy

Examination and assessment of the optic nerve (optic disc) and fundus with the direct ophthalmoscope or at the slit lamp with a non-contact or contact lens are essential to establish the diagnosis of open-angle glaucoma. (See 'The optic nerve in glaucoma' below for typical findings.)

Special tests

Elaborate and expensive examinations, such as tonography (measurement of rate of outflow of aqueous from the anterior chamber), ultrasonography (study of intraocular structures with ultrasound), and fluorescein angiography (study of intraocular blood vessels by intravenous fluorescein dye injection followed by special photography), may be possible only in tertiary eye centers or university medical schools. Most patients with primary open-angle glaucoma can be diagnosed without these special tests.

Chronic angle-closure glaucoma

History
Often silent; few symptoms. Occasionally aching pain may be present. Loss of peripheral vision may be noticeable in some patients. Loss of central visual acuity is a feature late in the process. If the angle closes suddenly, acute angle-closure glaucoma symptoms will likely be present.

Visual acuity
Central visual acuity is usually not lost or decreased until late in the disease.

Visual fields
Peripheral visual field loss may be present and can be demonstrated with perimetry.

Microscopic examination of the anterior segment
A clear cornea allows visual access to the anterior chamber. The anterior chamber is abnormally shallow. This can be determined by biomicroscopic examination or using a slit lamp or a flashlight (torch) by holding the light parallel with the iris from the temporal side – the oblique flashlight test (**70**).

Tonometry
Intraocular pressure is often mildly elevated. With an acute attack (360° closure), IOP may spike very high.

Gonioscopy
With a clear cornea, the drainage angle is partially occluded by peripheral anterior synechiae (PAS).

Ophthalmoscopy
Chronic elevated IOP at a level that cannot be tolerated by the eye will cause characteristic changes in the optic nerve head (optic disc), including increased cup/disc ratio, deepening of the cup, narrowing of the cup rim, notching, and paleness (pallor) of the disc.

70 Determining the depth of the anterior chamber using a flashlight: a) normal anterior chamber, b) shallow anterior chamber – a shadow is cast on the nasal iris.

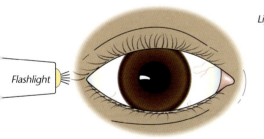

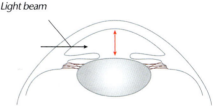

Light beam

a

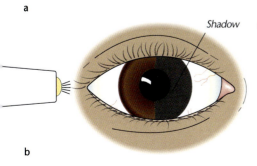

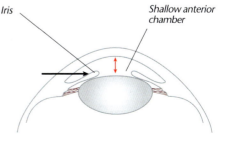

Shadow   Iris

Shallow anterior chamber

b

Acute angle-closure glaucoma

History

Pain, loss of vision and colored halos or rings around lights, usually in one eye, can be presenting complaints. Pain is often sudden and severe. Loss of vision may follow quickly because of corneal edema due to high IOP.

Visual acuity

Unlike primary open-angle glaucoma, central vision may be reduced suddenly and markedly in primary acute angle-closure glaucoma.

Visual fields

Visual field assessment is not possible or practical in an acute attack because of corneal edema causing poor visual acuity.

Microscopic examination of the anterior segment

Corneal clouding (due to edema) is present. The anterior chamber is shallow. The anterior chamber examination may be performed using a slit lamp, or by the oblique flashlight test (**70**). Cells and flare may be seen in the anterior chamber with the slit lamp. Subacute and chronic angle-closure glaucoma may not present with high pressure. These conditions may have minimal intraocular pressure elevation. The diagnosis may be suspected with the finding of a shallow anterior chamber as determined by the oblique flashlight test.

Tonometry

IOP is elevated, often to extremely high levels (50–60 mmHg). The eyeball will feel very firm with finger palpation over the upper eyelid.

Gonioscopy

Corneal edema may be present in an acute attack; NaCl 5% drops or ointment applied to the cornea may help clear corneal edema so that gonioscopy can be performed. In an acute attack, the normal angle structures cannot be seen with gonioscopy because the iris blocks the angle.

Ophthalmoscopy

This may not always be possible because of the presence of corneal edema, which will cause a poor view of the internal eye structures. In the early course of the disease, the optic disc is not severely damaged. Repeated attacks and chronic angle closure with elevated IOP will cause typical glaucoma damage to the optic disc.

Secondary glaucoma

History

The diagnosis of secondary glaucoma should be suspected if there is a history of injury to the eye, pain, and/or visual loss. Any penetrating injury or blunt trauma to the eye can cause secondary glaucoma. Diabetic patients, particularly those with neovascularization of the posterior segment structures, and any patient who has undergone intraocular surgery are secondary-glaucoma suspects. Secondary glaucomas are more often unilateral than primary open-angle glaucoma.

Tonometry

IOP measurements should always be performed in follow-up examinations of eyes that have been severely injured.

Childhood glaucoma

History

The parent or relative providing the history may describe tearing, enlargement of the eyes, corneal clouding, or apparent loss of vision.

Examination

The infant cornea and sclera are elastic and stretch with increased IOP, causing enlargement of the eyeball and resultant myopia. The horizontal diameter of the cornea of an eye with congenital glaucoma is greater than 11.5 mm. The enlarged eye in congenital glaucoma is called buphthalmos ('ox eye').

Tonometry

Examination under anesthesia should be done to accurately measure IOP. While the infant or child is under anesthesia, the pupils should be dilated and the optic nerve examined. The cup/disc ratio should be measured and the corneal diameters measured. Retinoscopy should also be performed.

Other tests

Gonioscopy and funduscopy under anesthesia should be done when congenital glaucoma is suspected. Even though congenital glaucoma is rare, the ophthalmic practitioner should be alert to the diagnosis in children. If medical and surgical management are neglected, the resulting blindness is irreversible. If there is doubt about the diagnosis, or if congenital glaucoma is suspected, the patient should be referred to a specialist for diagnosis and treatment.

The optic nerve in glaucoma

Many patients with primary open-angle glaucoma present themselves for treatment late in the disease, when the optic nerve is already severely and irreversibly damaged. Typical glaucomatous optic nerve damage includes the following:

- The normal central (physiological) optic cup in the center of the optic nerve deepens.
- Pinkish nerve tissue on the temporal side of the optic disc becomes damaged and thin, particularly in the inferior temporal optic disc quadrant. This is known as optic disc pallor.
- With uncontrolled glaucoma, the optic cup becomes pale, larger, and deeper. The optic cup enlarges and extends closer to the optic disc margins (**71**). A notch in the cup may occur. The notch will create a characteristic nerve fiber bundle defect that can be demonstrated on perimetry (see figure **67**).
- Tiny hemorrhages may appear on the optic disc.
- Optic nerve fibers in the optic disc are irreversibly damaged, causing characteristic visual field loss in glaucoma.

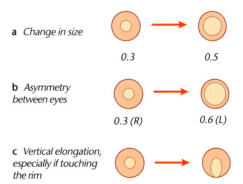

a *Change in size*

0.3   0.5

b *Asymmetry between eyes*

0.3 (R)   0.6 (L)

c *Vertical elongation, especially if touching the rim*

71 Suspect glaucoma if optic nerve cup increases in size over time (a), if there is asymmetry in size of the optic cup (b), or if the optic cup is not round and even (c).

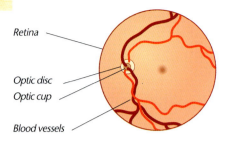

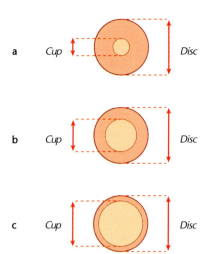

a   Cup   Disc

b   Cup   Disc

c   Cup   Disc

72 Cup/disc ratio. The normal diameter of the optic cup is 30% (or less) of the diameter of the optic disc; cup/disc ratio is 0.3 (a). In (b) the cup/disc ratio is 0.6: glaucoma is suspected. In (c) the cup/disc ratio is 0.9: glaucoma is responsible for damage to the optic disc.

The cup/disc ratio – the ratio of the optic cup in the vertical dimension to the total vertical optic disc dimension – is a useful examination measurement, observable by funduscopy (**72**). The normal cup/disc ratio is considered to be 3/10 (0.3) or less; in other words, 30% of the disc is cupped when measured vertically. In a cup/disc ratio greater than 3/10 (30%), glaucoma should be considered. Other measurements, especially tonometry and visual fields, should be performed to confirm the diagnosis. Making a sketch of the optic nerve cup at subsequent clinic visits will help to document change in progression in cup size and shape (**73**). This technique can help measure clinical change in the severity of glaucoma.

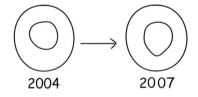

2004   2007

73 Drawing the appearance of the optic nerve cup, as seen in successive examinations, can be helpful in following the progression of glaucoma.

Visual fields in glaucoma

Peripheral vision can be lost in early glaucoma. The loss of peripheral vision is progressive, while central vision remains normal until late in the course of the disease. Together with a damaged optic disc, a constricted visual field can diagnose glaucoma. Elevated IOP above normal range (>21 mmHg) will confirm the diagnosis. If the visual field is constricted and the optic disc appears typically glaucomatous – but the IOP is normal – the patient likely has normotensive glaucoma.

The visual field can be measured by having the patient identify small test objects against a black felt cloth (a tangent screen). This formal testing of the visual field is called perimetry. Because it is a subjective test, the results are not reliable if the patient does not understand its purpose and is unable to cooperate.

Because perimetry is not usually available in rural ophthalmic practice settings, it is useful to be able to take an approximate visual field measurement with cross-confrontation visual-field testing (see algorithm, above right).

Although ophthalmic health care workers in major ophthalmic referral centers should learn formal visual-field testing, cross-confrontation field testing may be taught to rural eye care workers by an experienced ophthalmic practitioner. Cross-confrontation fields can provide valuable additional information to assist in establishing a diagnosis of glaucoma.

Medical management

Current accepted management of glaucoma is to control IOP and lower it to a level at which damage to the optic nerve and retina is stopped. Medical and surgical management can lower IOP and stop progression of peripheral visual field loss.

Primary open-angle glaucoma may be managed medically and/or surgically. Primary acute angle-closure glaucoma is usually managed by surgical intervention after controlling the pain and elevated IOP by medical means. Secondary glaucomas are managed both medically and surgically. Infantile glaucoma requires immediate medical and surgical management in early life to prevent blindness.

Medical management is the more conservative method of managing glaucoma but often is not practical for long-term treatment. (See also the closing comments in this chapter.) Because glaucoma is a chronic disease that medications do not cure, several conditions must be met for medical management to be effective:

- Medications must be readily available and inexpensive.
- The patient must have access to a medical treatment center where tonometry may be performed and the patient examined at regular intervals.
- The patient with glaucoma must understand fully the necessity of using the prescribed medications regularly and indefinitely on a daily basis and must be cooperative and reliable in using them. Instruction in placing drops in eyes is usually necessary. The patient must understand also that eye drops will not restore vision but can only control pressure to preserve existing vision if used properly.
- The eye health care worker must be skilled and very attentive in the diagnosis and medical management of glaucoma.
- For blindness to be prevented, the patient must be followed by trained ophthalmic practitioners at regular intervals.

Medications used to lower intraocular pressure

This section discusses the major groups of drugs used to control high IOP, along with their benefits and side effects. Severe systemic complications can result from long-term use of medications used to lower IOP. Therapy has to be planned and managed carefully. Some of these drugs may not be relevant in certain areas of the developing world because of shortages, non-availability, or prohibitively high cost.

Miotics

Miotics cause miosis, or constriction of the pupil. They are also called parasympathomimetics because they produce effects similar to those produced by stimulation of the parasympathetic nerves. These medications act to drain aqueous more rapidly through the trabecular meshwork in the angle.

The miotic pilocarpine is the most widely available and least expensive medication for the medical control of glaucoma. Pilocarpine is available in 1–6% solutions (6% pilocarpine is impractical for outpatient use, however, because of side effects). The dosage is one drop topically every 6 hours. Side effects can include visual disturbances, blurring, frontal headache, and nausea, and patients often stop using pilocarpine because of them.

Echothiophate iodide, a long-term miotic, is given every 12 hours, but side effects are greater than with pilocarpine. This medication is not frequently used.

Miotics such as pilocarpine should be discontinued for patients awaiting cataract surgery. The miotic pupil created by these drugs makes cataract surgery difficult. The patient should be switched to another type of IOP-lowering medication pre-operatively.

Miotics will congest and further inflame already inflamed eyes. They should not be used in glaucoma secondary to neovascularization of diabetes mellitus. Likewise, they should not be used to control high IOP when the anterior segment is inflamed, as in uveitis.

Epinephrine

Epinephrine is a sympathomimetic because it mimics the action of sympathetic nerves in the eye. The drug acts to reduce the volume of aqueous produced by the ciliary body. Epinephrine has a minor dilating effect on the pupil. Epinephrine hydrochloride 1% solution is administered one drop every 8 hours to the affected eye. It causes a stinging sensation when applied topically to the eye; patients often find instillation uncomfortable and stop using it.

Epinephrine is contraindicated in patients with heart disease and high blood pressure. Because refrigeration is required to maintain its strength, epinephrine is impractical in regions where electricity and refrigeration are unavailable. Topical epinephrine hydrochloride 1% solution is useful preoperatively to cause vasoconstriction of conjunctival vessels and a resulting dry operating field for intraocular surgery.

Beta blockers

The beta blockers (beta-adrenergic blocking agents) reduce the production of aqueous by the ciliary body. Timolol maleate was the first of the beta blockers to be developed for the treatment of glaucoma and ocular hypertension. Timolol maleate and most other drugs in this class are administered one drop every 12 hours to the affected eye(s), although once-daily use is effective in up to 70% of patients.

Beta blockers generally have little effect on the pupil and are usually excellent medications for lowering IOP. They are expensive, however, making them impractical for widespread long-term use in the developing world. Beta blockers are contraindicated in congestive heart failure, asthma, and chronic lung disease.

Carbonic anhydrase inhibitors

Drugs in this group lower IOP by reducing aqueous production by the ciliary body. Acetazolamide is a carbonic anhydrase inhibitor that is widely available in oral form. The dose is one 250-mg tablet every 6 hours for an adult. Acetazolamide 500-mg sequels may be given orally every 12 hours. A topical acetazolamide preparation is also available, but for maximum effect, it must be applied three times a day to the affected eyes.

Serious side effects from acetazolamide can occur. The drug should not be used for long-term treatment. Systemic side effects include formation of kidney stones, disturbances in body chemistry, and gastrointestinal disturbances. Patients frequently suffer loss of appetite and weight loss. Potassium is lost from the body with long-term use of acetazolamide, contributing to heart-rhythm disturbances. Eating one banana per day will replace the potassium lost due to the drug; fortunately, bananas are abundant and inexpensive in most tropical nations.

Acetazolamide is expensive. This factor and its side effects make it a poor choice for outpatient management of glaucoma. Acetazolamide is useful in the hospital setting, however, to lower IOP prior to surgery and to control acute angle-closure glaucoma. Methazolamide is another oral carbonic anhydrase inhibitor that is similar in efficacy and side effects to acetazolamide.

Hyperosmotics

Glycerin (called also glycerol) is an oral medication that dehydrates vitreous to lower IOP. It is not expensive, it is easy to give to patients, and it is widely available. It may be used to assist in breaking an acute attack of angle-closure glaucoma.

Mannitol and urea are intravenous hyperosmotics that are expensive and not widely available. Hyperosmotic agents are usually reserved for hospital use and have little role in outpatient glaucoma management (dosing is difficult to manage because they are liquids).

Prostaglandin inhibitors

Latanoprost, a prostaglandin agent that lowers IOP by increasing outflow through a pathway other than the trabecular meshwork, is a topical medication that is used once a day in the affected eyes. Prostaglandin agents are instilled in affected eyes at night because the maximum effect of the drug occurs approximately 12 hours later, or when intraocular pressures are highest in human eyes. These drugs require refrigeration to maintain potency and are expensive, both disadvantages in rural areas of the developing world. The advantages are that there are few side effects, the drug is quite safe, and it is used only once a day, at night.

Alpha-adrenergic agonists

Apraclonidine and brimonidine are alpha-adrenergic agonists that decrease aqueous production and thus IOP when applied topically. Both drugs (especially apraclonidine) may be associated with a high rate of allergic reactions. Do not administer these drugs to very elderly people or to children.

Primary acute angle-closure glaucoma

In an acute attack of primary angle-closure glaucoma, medical therapy should be started as soon as possible to lower IOP and to prevent damage to the eye and loss of vision. If IOP is >50 mmHg, administer IV mannitol to first lower intraocular pressure before surgically entering the eye. Mannitol dosage must be calculated according to the weight of the patient. Once the IOP is lowered and the acute attack has been broken, a surgical iridectomy or iridotomy must be undertaken as soon as possible (see below).

Immediate medical treatment consists of one or more of the following regimens:

- Miotic: one drop of pilocarpine 4% every 30 min until the pupil constricts.
- Beta blocker: one drop of timolol maleate 0.5% every 10 min until the IOP is reduced to within normal range.
- Carbonic anhydrase inhibitor: one dose of acetazolamide 500 mg orally.
- Hyperosmotic: glycerin 50% solution given orally, 1.5 g per kilogram of body weight.
- Hypermostic IV if possible (mannitol, as described above).

Pain in end-stage glaucoma

Pain often appears late in glaucoma when IOP is very high (40–50 mmHg or higher). The discomfort and pain may be managed by controlling the IOP with pilocarpine (if the eye is not inflamed or irritated) or with timolol maleate, although this is expensive long-term treatment. Pilocarpine should not be used (contraindicated) to treat high intraocular pressure if the eye is inflamed (rubeosis, uveitis, iritis, scleritis, and conjunctivitis).

Pain from end-stage glaucoma may also be permanently alleviated with retrobulbar 90% alcohol; 1 ml of 90% alcohol is injected together with 2 ml of local anesthetic (1% lidocaine, for example) behind the eye. If pain is not controlled with retrobulbar alcohol, the blind and painful eye should be enucleated (removed surgically).

Surgical management

Surgery to lower IOP should be performed when medical management fails or is not practical. Like medical management, surgery can only stop further visual loss; it cannot restore vision already lost from glaucoma. Surgery for glaucoma should be undertaken if the patient has useful vision that can be maintained by permanently lowering IOP. (See Appendix D for a list of equipment and supplies useful for performing glaucoma surgery; see Appendix C for glaucoma surgery guidelines for ophthalmic medical auxiliaries.)

Filtration surgery

A variety of external filtration operations have been developed for surgical management of primary open-angle glaucoma. Filtration surgery may also be performed on certain secondary glaucomas. Filtration operations attempt to establish a permanent fistula (opening) from the anterior chamber to the subconjunctival space. The filtration operation creates a new outflow pathway and bypasses the blocked trabecular meshwork. The IOP can then return to normal, and damage to the optic nerve and retina can be stopped. As with cataract surgery, there are certain risks with glaucoma filtration surgery. The risks include external infection, scarring of the surgical site and failure of the operation, secondary cataract, phthisis bulbi, and endophthalmitis.

Trabeculectomy is the most commonly performed external filtration operation. A tiny block of sclera and trabecular meshwork at the limbus is removed, with the opening covered by a loosely sutured scleral flap. Aqueous flows through this fistula to the subconjunctival space, creating a bleb (a small rounded mound). If the trabeculectomy functions well, IOP becomes normal because of constant aqueous outflow through the fistula.

An iridectomy (removal of a tiny piece of peripheral iris) is usually performed during the trabeculectomy operation. The iridectomy creates a channel from the anterior chamber to the posterior chamber. A fistula is created over the iridectomy through the resected sclera. Trabeculectomy and iridectomy may be performed under local anesthesia using cataract instruments. Trabeculectomy is considered safer than other filtration operations in which only conjunctiva covers the fistula opening. There are fewer postoperative complications following trabeculectomy.

Filtration operations frequently fail in darkly pigmented people. The fistula closes by scarring and then ceases to function, causing IOP to rise. Antimetabolite drugs, including 5-fluorouracil and mitomycin C, can be used at the time of filtration surgery to delay healing of the scleral opening. Antimetabolites, if used in the proper dosage and with care at the time of surgery, can increase the rate of success of filtration surgery, but they may also cause several serious complications such as scleral melting, delayed healing, wound leak, endophthalmitis, and prolonged low IOP (hypotony). Antimetabolites in glaucoma filtration surgery should be used only by experienced intraocular surgeons.

Iridectomy and iridotomy in acute primary angle-closure glaucoma

In an acute attack of primary angle-closure glaucoma, the anterior chamber is shallow, the pupil is in mid-dilation, and the angle and trabecular meshwork are obstructed. The passage of aqueous fluid through the pupil into the anterior chamber is blocked at the lens and iris, a condition known as pupillary block. (See Figure 165 for a diagram of the normal flow of aqueous.) Adhesions between the iris and the lens (posterior synechiae) may form if the pupillary block is not broken (**74**).

If total 360° posterior synechiae form, aqueous can push the iris forward, a condition known as iris bombé (**75**). Posterior synechiae from uveitis can have the same result. An opening between the anterior chamber and the posterior chamber must be made with a surgical opening in the iris (iridectomy) or argon laser (iridotomy) in order to break the pupillary block and to allow aqueous to enter the anterior chamber.

After the IOP has been controlled medically in an acute attack of angle-closure glaucoma, surgical peripheral iridectomy in the operating room is the definitive treatment to establish this new anterior chamber/posterior chamber

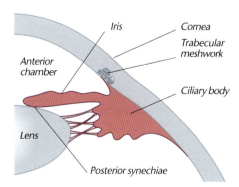

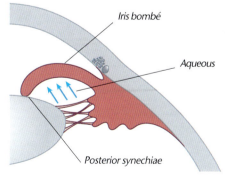

74 Posterior synechiae, in which the iris adheres to the lens (see also Figure 152).

75 Iris bombé, in which the iris is forced forward when posterior synechiae block aqueous from entering the anterior chamber.

opening. There is no external fistula created in this operation. The operation can be performed under local anesthesia. Alternatively, an opening in the peripheral iris may be created with an argon or Nd:YAG laser (iridotomy) without doing a surgical operation. Lasers may be available at tertiary eye centers.

A prophylactic surgical iridectomy or laser iridotomy must be done in the fellow eye in a patient who has required surgery to break an angle-closure attack. If a prophylactic iridectomy or iridotomy is not done in the fellow eye, the eye will likely sustain an acute angle-closure attack later.

Special considerations

Management of secondary glaucoma

Secondary glaucoma may be managed either medically or surgically. Medical management is possible only if the general conditions for medical management are met (see above); it can be complicated and difficult. Systemic causes of secondary glaucoma must be controlled (diabetes, for example, may be the cause of neovascular glaucoma). Local causes of secondary glaucoma must also be corrected (hyphema, for example, may block and damage the angle).

Secondary glaucoma can be caused by an advanced cataract or dislocated lens. Phacomorphic glaucoma results when the lens increases in size with age (hypermature cataract), pushes the iris forward, and blocks the angle. Cataract extraction will usually relieve the blocked angle and lower the IOP.

Phacolytic glaucoma results when a hypermature cataract leaks liquefied lens material into the anterior chamber, causing uveitis and glaucoma. The inflammation and acute IOP rise should be controlled medically and the cataract removed as soon as possible (see Chapter 5).

Contusion or blunt injury to the eye can produce a luxated (dislocated) or sub-luxated (partially dislocated) lens. Secondary glaucoma may result. Post-traumatic glaucoma secondary to contusion injury may be managed medically or surgically, depending on indications.

Intraocular inflammation and secondary glaucoma

If uveitis is present with glaucoma, the etiology should be determined, if possible (see Chapter 12), and the systemic disease related to uveitis should be treated appropriately. Uveitis should be managed with corticosteroids and topical atropine 1%.

Intraocular inflammation should be controlled before intraocular surgery (cataract extraction or filtration surgery for glaucoma) is performed. Surgery on an inflamed eye may result in phthisis bulbi (shrinkage and atrophy of the eye).

Peripheral anterior synechiae (PAS), or adhesions between the peripheral iris and the cornea, may result from chronic inflammation or repeated attacks of angle-closure glaucoma (**76**). These synechiae cannot be surgically lysed to restore normal function.

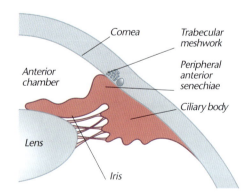

76 Peripheral anterior synechiae, in which the iris occludes the trabecular meshwork.

Neovascular glaucoma

Neovascular glaucoma is a form of glaucoma caused by neovascularization of the iris and anterior chamber angle. Tips on its management are as follows:

- Medical management often fails. Miotics should be avoided as they may further congest the eye.
- Cyclocryopexy (freezing a portion of the ciliary body through the sclera) can reduce aqueous production and lower IOP. A locally manufactured cryosurgery instrument (see Chapter 3) may be used.
- Newer Nd:YAG and diode lasers make it possible to more precisely destroy the ciliary body, thereby decreasing IOP.
- Filtration surgery may be possible but frequently fails.

Cataract and glaucoma

The rate of occurrence of cataract and primary glaucoma, particularly primary open-angle glaucoma, increases progressively with age. Cataract and glaucoma may occur at the same time in the same eye.

Glaucoma filtration surgery and cataract extraction can be performed at the same time when both conditions are present. Trabeculectomy is the safest filtration procedure in this regard. The trabeculectomy is done before extracting the cataract, and the corneoscleral incision is repaired so as to leave a fistula and filtering bleb.

Cataract extraction and cyclodialysis, an 'internal filtering' operation, are sometimes performed together in patients with open-angle glaucoma and cataract. In this case, a curved spatula is inserted through the angle posteriorly against the sclera. The spatula is moved from side to side to separate sclera from choroid to form a cleft in the angle for drainage of aqueous. Although this is a time-saving glaucoma operation, it is risky because of possible hemorrhage from the choroid. Extensive bleeding from the choroid and loss of intraocular contents (expulsive choroidal hemorrhage) may occur at the time of surgery, and hyphema is a frequent postoperative complication.

Prevention of blindness from glaucoma

Prevention of blindness from glaucoma, particularly primary open-angle glaucoma, is difficult because many patients present very late for treatment after extensive damage to the optic nerve has already occurred and peripheral vision has been permanently lost. Although primary open-angle glaucoma cannot be prevented, further deterioration of vision can be arrested in patients who have already sustained visual loss.

Early diagnosis

Successful management of glaucoma depends on early diagnosis. The eye health care worker should always suspect glaucoma, particularly in adults. Tonometry should be performed on all adults and all patients at high risk of developing glaucoma (diabetics and people of African descent, for example). Since primary open-angle glaucoma can be familial, relatives of these patients should be carefully examined. The fundus and optic disc should be examined in all adults.

Early surgery

The cost of a lifetime of medications used in outpatient management of primary open-angle glaucoma is great. Patients often live far from treatment facilities, even mobile eye units, and cannot be examined regularly. Generally, patient cooperation in glaucoma medical management is poor.

Patients usually do not understand the natural history of glaucoma. Most expect medical management to improve vision.

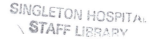

When vision does not improve with medical therapy, they lose faith in the treatment. They stop taking the medication and fail to return for follow-up care.

Early filtration surgery is recommended in primary open-angle glaucoma patients who will almost certainly become medical management failures. This recommendation is opposite to glaucoma practice in industrialized countries, where surgery for primary open-angle glaucoma is performed only after medical and laser management have failed.

Infantile glaucoma surgery may be performed to lower IOP at an early age. Either goniotomy (incising the congenital tissue that is blocking the angle) or trabeculectomy is the operation of choice.

7

Trachoma

Trachoma is an immense subject, in the literature replete with hypotheses, discussions, and polemics, in the world pregnant with suffering disability and blindness. Its importance as a source of human suffering and as a national economic loss over large tracts of the world's surface is second to none among the diseases of the eye, or, indeed, among diseases of all kinds.
Sir Stewart Duke-Elder

Trachoma is a chronic keratoconjunctivitis caused by the bacterium *Chlamydia trachomatis* that primarily affects the superior and inferior tarsal conjunctiva and cornea. The term 'trachoma' is derived from a Greek word meaning 'rough,' which describes the appearance and irregularity of the conjunctiva with acute trachomatous infection. It is a disease of poor hygiene and poverty. If not treated, trachoma infection can result in blindness or low vision. Trachoma control can be achieved by improving sanitation, providing clean water, and treating individuals and communities with appropriate antibiotics. Correction of entropion and trichiasis (**77**) is possible through eyelid surgery. This chapter discusses the epidemiology, clinical diagnosis and management of trachoma. Public health measures currently applied in trachoma control are presented.

Epidemiology

Trachoma is one of the most common diseases in the world. Although it is localized in distribution and is declining in both incidence and prevalence, it remains a significant cause of blindness worldwide. The World Health Organization (WHO) in 2002 estimated that nearly 4% of all blind people (1,350,000 people) were blind from trachoma. The rates of active infection are declining because of the implementation of the SAFE strategy (described in this chapter), improved hygiene, public health education, and national campaigns.

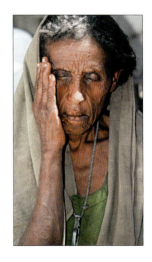

77 Ethiopian woman with entropion and trichiasis. Note tweezers on necklace for eyelash epilation.

2 Regions and countries of the world where trachoma remains a major cause of external ocular disease, low vision, and blindness include:

- Africa: countries of western, eastern, and southern Africa and the Horn of Africa, Sudan.
- Mediterranean and Middle East: Morocco, Tunisia, Libya, Egypt, Djibouti, Saudi Arabia, the Gulf states, Iran, Afghanistan, Pakistan.
- Asia: India, Nepal, Myanmar, China.
- Southeast Asia and western Pacific: Laos, Vietnam, Philippines, Australia, and some Pacific islands.
- Americas: Mexico, Guatemala, Brazil, Bolivia, Peru.

Trachoma is a disease of overcrowded and unclean living environments. It is spread from person to person and from eye to eye by poor hygiene and contaminated fingers. Dirty linen, contaminated water, substandard body hygiene, inadequate latrines, and house flies are implicated (**78**). Flies seek the moisture of mucous membranes (the conjunctivae, in this case) in dry climates and probably spread the *Chlamydia* bacterium from person to person. Trachoma is a cluster disease,

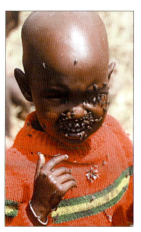

78 Active trachoma and moisture seeking flies. Trachoma begins in childhood in endemic regions.

meaning that in crowded family and community groups where trachoma is present, most people tend to be affected by the disease. In a community where trachoma is endemic, family groups with good hygiene may be unaffected or the disease may be present only in a mild form. People most severely affected by trachoma are usually infected early in childhood and remain infected most of their lives. Repeated reinfection throughout life can result in blindness, hence the term 'blinding trachoma'. Blinding trachoma can be prevented by breaking the cycle of reinfection by interrupting the transmission of the *Chlamydia trachomatis* bacterium. Blindness from trichiasis secondary to trachoma can be prevented by performing trichiasis surgery as soon as entropion with trichiasis is diagnosed.

Other factors that influence the severity and chronicity of trachoma in individuals, families, and communities include:

- Standard of living.
- Availability and use of clean water for face washing.
- Use of sanitary latrines.
- Access to and use of health treatment facilities (**79**).
- Availability and proper use of medications used for treating trachoma.
- Level of education and awareness of patients and the community.

Infection with trachoma confers little or no immunity. A patient once cured of active trachoma may be reinfected at any time. Chronic trachoma may be assumed by the patient and the community to be a natural condition of childhood. A child with trachoma may not be examined by an eye health care worker as a result, and the disease and cycle of reinfection may not be broken if the child remains infected.

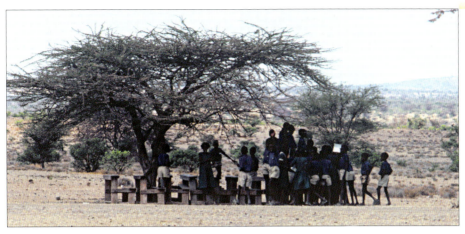

79 Screening villagers in an endemic trachoma area.

Clinical diagnosis

Trachoma should be suspected in any patient with external ocular infection who lives or has lived in a region of the world where the disease is endemic.

In order to diagnose trachoma accurately, the tarsal conjunctiva must be examined. The examiner must evert both upper eyelids. A 2.5-power loupe and a bright flashlight (torch) will make possible an accurate examination of the tarsal conjunctiva and are needed for grading the disease. The normal conjunctiva of the upper tarsal area is smooth, thin, transparent, and has a pinkish appearance. Large blood vessels in the tarsal conjunctiva are positioned vertically from the upper and lower edges of the tarsal plate.

The eyelids should also be examined carefully for evidence of in-turned eyelashes. The cornea should be examined for vascularization and corneal opacity (nebula, macula, or leukoma).

Trachoma is nearly always bilateral. The infection begins in the upper tarsal conjunctiva but also involves the inferior fornix. Papillae (tiny blood vessel tufts) and

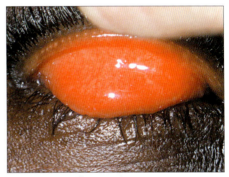

80 Intense papillary reaction.

widespread papillary reaction in the conjunctivae are initial responses to infection. Papillary reaction gives a diffuse, bright red appearance to the conjunctiva if acute infection is present (**80**).

The presence of follicles (follicular reaction) of the conjunctiva also indicates that acute infection is present. Follicles are whitish isolated elevations within the conjunctiva, especially the tarsal conjunctiva.

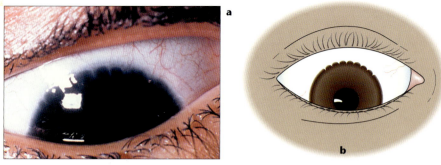

81 Herbert's pits at limbus, characteristic of chronic trachoma: clinical appearence (a); location (b).

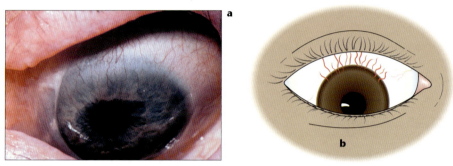

82 Vascular pannus in inflammatory trachoma: clinical appearence (a); location (b).

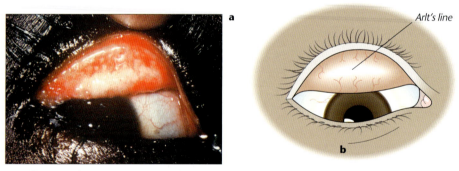

83 Chronic trachoma resulting in papillary reaction, follicles, and Arlt's line (a). Arlt's line (b).

Follicles also occur at the limbus, particularly at the superior limbus, and when healed leave characteristic scars, known as Herbert's pits (**81**). These small, round limbal scars are characteristic only of past trachoma infection and of spontaneous healing with scarring.

Each follicle is a small accumulation of acute and chronic inflammatory cells,

discharge, and some *Chlamydia* bacteria. The bacteria multiply in conjunctival epithelial cells and are released into the tear film when the cells are broken down. The fresh *Chlamydia* bacteria may reinfect the conjunctiva or infect the conjunctivae of other people if transmitted through poor hygiene or a vector (unclean clothing or the house fly).

Acute infection can result in downward blood vessel growth over the limbus and onto the cornea (pannus) in the superior fornices and superior globe (**82**). Vascular pannus can scar the cornea and can extend to cover the visual axis and produce a corneal nebula or corneal macula, resulting in visual disability or blindness. *Chlamydia* infection of the corneal epithelium produces a punctate staining pattern with fluorescein (punctate keratitis).

More follicles rupture as the infection worsens. When healing occurs, scarring and shrinkage result, particularly in the superior tarsal conjunctiva. Scarring of the conjunctiva varies in severity. A severe horizontal scar of the upper tarsal conjunctiva is known as Arlt's line (**83**).

Severe conjunctival scarring causes shortening of the tarsal plate and in-turning of the eyelid margin (entropion). Conjunctival scarring also occurs in the inferior fornices but rarely causes entropion. When entropion of the upper eyelid is severe, eyelashes are turned inward and touch and abrade the cornea, a condition known as trichiasis (**84**). The eyelid margin may be distorted from tarsal shortening due to scarring, resulting in curving of the eyelid margin.

Chronic trichiasis is often accompanied by secondary bacterial infection and ulceration of the cornea. Corneal abrasions due to trichiasis predispose the individual to bacterial invasion and ulceration.

A corneal ulcer, when healed, may produce a potentially blinding white scar (leukoma).

Almost any bacterium can cause secondary infection. Ulceration of the cornea is a risk of bacterial keratoconjunctivitis. The following bacterial pathogens are among the most common causes:

- *Streptococcus pneumoniae* (*Diplococcus* and *Pneumococcus* are other names in use).
- *Staphylococcus*.
- *Moraxella* (Morax–Axenfeld bacillus).
- *Haemophilus aegyptius* (Koch–Weeks bacillus) – a rare cause of central corneal ulceration; a more common cause of marginal ulcers in endemic trachoma areas where seasonal conjunctivitis is a common occurrence.

If not treated and controlled, corneal ulceration secondary to trichiasis may result in corneal perforation and endophthalmitis. Multiple infections must occur before trachoma results in entropion, trichiasis, corneal scarring, perforation, and blindness.

Trachoma, together with secondary infection and sometimes vitamin A deficiency in children, may also cause weakening and stretching of corneal tissue and places the eye with trachoma at higher risk of corneal ulceration from this mechanism as well. The cornea and iris bulge forward, producing a staphyloma. Chronic trachomatous and/or bacterial infection of the lacrimal sac(s), *dacryocystitis*, may occur with trachoma infection. Finally, chronic scarring of the conjunctiva can produce *symblepharon*, or adhesions of the tarsal conjunctiva to the bulbar conjunctiva.

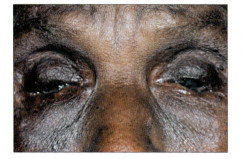

84 Bilateral severe end-stage trachoma with entropion and trichiasis.

Grading system

In 1987, the World Health Organization developed a simplified grading system for trachoma. The area of tarsal conjunctiva to be examined is indicated in **85**. The system is based on the presence or absence of the following five key signs:

- Trachomatous inflammation – follicular (TF).
- Trachomatous inflammation – intense, or papillary (TI).
- Trachomatous scarring (TS).
- Trachomatous trichiasis (TT).
- Corneal opacity (CO).

Each type of inflammation may vary in intensity, and both follicular and papillary inflammation may occur together (**86**). The following list gives the classic findings and implications of each grade:

- TF (trachomatous inflammation – follicular). The presence of five or more follicles in the upper tarsal conjunctiva (**84, 87**); implies significant active disease and should be treated with antibiotics.
- TI (trachomatous inflammation – intense). Pronounced inflammatory thickening of the upper tarsal conjunctiva that obscures more than half of the normal deep tarsal vessels (**88**). Intense papillary reaction causes the tarsal plate conjunctiva to appear red and smooth (**89**). Follicles in the conjunctiva may be obscured; implies intense active disease and is in need of treatment and careful surveillance; this is the future high-risk group for trachomatous blindness (**90**).

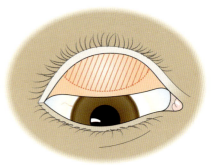

85 Everted eyelid shows the area of tarsal conjunctiva (shaded) to be examined for assessment of trachoma.

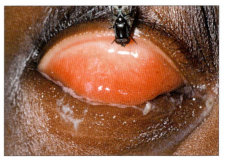

86 Inflammatory trachoma and scarring (TI, TF, and TS).

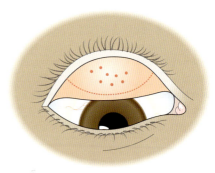

87 Trachomatous inflammation – follicular (TF).

- TS (trachomatous scarring). The presence of scarring in the tarsal conjunctiva. Scars may appear as fine white lines in the tarsal conjunctiva. Diffuse scarring will appear as a whitish fibrous area or patch. This should not be confused with inflammatory thickening; implies the presence of scarring, indicating present or previous inflammatory disease. Arlt's line (**90**) is a dense scar that frequently results in entropion with trichiasis.
- TT (trachomatous trichiasis). At least one eyelash rubs on the eyeball. If the eyelash has been epilated (pulled out) or cut off close to the eyelid margin, the condition is still graded as trichiasis; implies trichiasis in need of surgery; a potentially disabling condition.

- CO (corneal opacity). Easily visible corneal opacity over the pupil. Corneal opacity is graded if a corneal scar extends over the pupil and causes the pupillary margin to be blurred when viewed through the opacity (**91**). Visual acuity should always be measured in patients with corneal scarring because the corneal opacity can cause significant visual impairment (less than 6/18 [20/60] visual acuity); implies corneal opacity due to trachoma; potentially disabling or blinding.

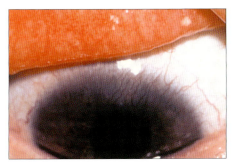

88 inflammatory trachoma (TI) and vascular pannus.

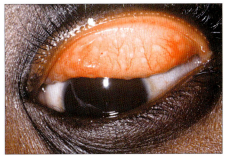

89 Inflammatory trachoma, TI and TF.

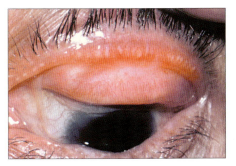

90 Arlt's line (TS) and trachomatous infection of Meibomian glands (WHO).

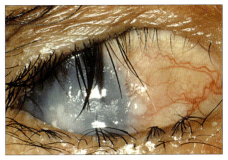

91 Chronic entropion and trichiasis resulting in leukoma (CO) from corneal ulceration.

Medical management of trachoma

Topical antibiotics

The tetracycline drugs (tetracycline, oxytetracycline, and chlortetracycline) are inexpensive and widely available. Tetracycline as 1% ointment or in oily suspension is the preferred drug for topical treatment of active trachoma. (Topical erythromycin, although not as effective as tetracycline in treating trachoma, may be substituted if topical tetracycline is not available.)

For acute and active trachoma, the WHO recommends tetracycline 1% ointment or suspension applied to both eyes three times daily (every 8 hours) for at least 6 weeks. Treatment with tetracycline should be accompanied by face washing with soap and water, if possible, or with clean water alone if soap is not available.

Family and community-based intermittent topical treatment with tetracycline can form the basis of trachoma control in severely affected communities. The recommended WHO intermittent treatment schedule consists of applications of tetracycline 1% ointment or suspension to both eyes twice daily (every 12 hours) for 5 consecutive days each month, or once daily for 10 days each month and for at least 6 consecutive months each year. This schedule may be repeated as often as necessary.

Systemic antibiotics

As topical sulfonamides are only moderately effective against trachoma, oral sulfonamides used to be administered in therapeutic doses to treat active trachoma. Because a severe and sometimes fatal systemic reaction (Stevens–Johnson syndrome) can follow the administration of a sulfonamide drug, this treatment is no longer recommended or used to treat trachoma.

Oral tetracycline can be effective against trachoma, but because of side effects, it should usually be given only to children over 6–8 years of age and to adult males and non-pregnant women. Side effects may include staining of teeth, retarded bone growth, and adverse effects on the fetus in pregnant women.

Azithromycin (an azalide) is a new antibiotic that has shown great promise in treating trachoma. It appears to be very effective against *Chlamydia trachomatis* when given to adults in a one-time 1-g dose. Azithromycin appears to have few serious adverse side effects and may be used in children older than age 6 months. This drug may have an important role in coming years in the community control of trachoma and in the possible eradication of this disease.

Surgical management of entropion and trichiasis

For eyelids with entropion and trichiasis (**92**), surgery should be performed to correct the deformity and to prevent further damage to the cornea. There is no need to operate on entropion if trichiasis is not present. Surgical strategies include epilation, electrolysis, cryoablation, and trichiasis surgery. Trichiasis surgery is the preferred method of correcting entropion with trichiasis.

Epilation

Patients may themselves remove individual eyelashes with tweezers or forceps. This is not an appropriate strategy for severe trichiasis but may work for minor cases. If the eyelashes grow back, they may be firm and stiff, and may cause further damage to the cornea.

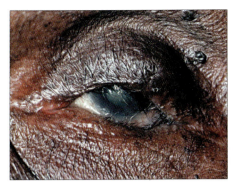

92 Marked entropion and trichiasis secondary to trachoma in an adult.

Electrolysis

In electrolysis, the root (follicle) of the eyelash is destroyed with low-voltage electrical current. This method is more complicated than simple epilation. Fine-wire probes and an electric power source are necessary. Removed eyelashes may recur.

Cryoablation

In cryoablation, the eyelash follicle(s) is/are destroyed using a cryoextractor tip that operates at below-freezing temperatures for an extended time. Results may not be as good as simple epilation.

Trichiasis surgery

Surgical technicians may be trained to perform these operations by ophthalmologists familiar with the techniques. This surgery may be performed under local anesthesia at a community clinic in a clean operating room. The affected upper eyelids should be corrected surgically as soon as possible.

Many different procedures for entropion with trichiasis have been devised; none of the procedures will be successful in all surgeries. Entropion with trichiasis may recur months to years after the surgery depending on how much scarring of the tarsal plate was present and which procedure was performed.

The most successful operation (the one with the lowest recurrence rate) seems to be the bilamellar tarsal rotation procedure. This is the operation recommended by the World Health Organization. The technique, equipment, and supplies needed to perform this operation are described in the WHO booklet *Trichiasis Surgery for Trachoma: The Bilamellar Tarsal Rotation Procedure*, listed in Appendix I.

Public health and trachoma

Trachoma should be controlled at the community level. Trachoma may disappear when the standard of living in the community improves significantly. A successful trachoma control program depends on the availability of ample clean water for washing and good personal hygiene (**93**). To ensure success, a comprehensive community trachoma control program should be coordinated with community water development and construction of sanitary latrines.

Public health and hygiene education for everyone in an affected community – children and adults – is necessary for a

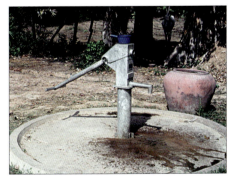

93 A borehole provides clean and safe water for cooking, drinking, and hygiene. Regular face washing with uncontaminated water is essential for trachoma control.

successful control program. Public health education for prevention of disease can be carried out in schools and community centers. Early diagnosis through mass screening programs will identify individual patients, family groups, and communities to be treated; however, mass treatment campaigns by themselves for eradication of trachoma are not effective without improvement in the community standard of living and better hygienic practices. Promotion of trichiasis surgery is also a key element of a successful trachoma control program. Case identification of patients with trichiasis is essential. Trichiasis surgery should be available to all those patients who require it.

SAFE strategy

For hygiene promotion, blindness prevention, and community support, the SAFE strategy is recommended:

S – surgery for trichiasis
A – antibiotics to treat inflammatory disease
F – face washing, particularly in children
E – environmental changes, including provision of clean water and improvement of household sanitation.

The SAFE strategy requires the coordination and participation of health care workers, community leaders, and individuals, households, and communities affected by trachoma.

GET 2020

In 1996, an alliance for the Global Elimination of Trachoma was formed between many non-governmental organizations dedicated to the prevention of blindness, private foundations, ministries of health, and the World Health Organization Program for the Prevention of Blindness and Deafness. The goal of the alliance is the eradication of trachoma by the year 2020 (GET 2020).

GET 2020 is an important component of Vision 2020, an international and global initiative to reduce both the prevalence and incidence of blindness and low vision.

Ocular trauma

*Insufficient medical facilities or trained personnel make ocular trauma
a serious threat to vision in much of the world.*
International Agency for the Prevention of Blindness, 1980

O cular trauma is a major cause of monocular blindness but is less often responsible for bilateral blindness. Accurate diagnosis and prompt treatment of eye injuries are essential to prevent blindness. Trauma takes many forms. This chapter classifies eye injuries both by type of injury (e.g., contusion, laceration, intraocular foreign body) and by anatomic location (injury to eyelids, ocular surface injury). The chapter also discusses harmful eye practices of traditional healers and the devastating international problems of antipersonnel landmines (94).

General considerations

All ocular injuries are considered to be emergencies and should be treated promptly. Immediate referral of any ocular injury is necessary if the health care worker who examines the patient initially is unable to treat the injury. Seemingly minor injuries to the eye, such as corneal abrasion, may become infected and result in serious corneal damage, loss of vision, and even blindness if not managed correctly. Thorough ocular examination is vital (see Chapter 16). Note the following:

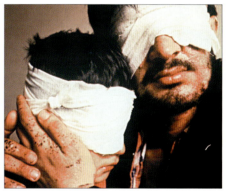

94 Middle Eastern father and son with ocular injuries from landmine explosion.

- Visual acuity should be measured if possible.
- Topical anesthesia drops may facilitate examination, especially when it is necessary to retract the eyelids.
- Low intraocular pressure (hypotony) may indicate ocular penetration.

- Foreign body penetration into the intraocular space may have occurred.
- Fluorescein dye will reveal corneal abrasion and epithelial defects (see Figure 167).

See *Table 6* for a list of common causes of ocular injuries.

Patching

Patching the eye serves a specific purpose: it 'splints' the upper eyelid over the cornea to put the eye at rest. If further protection is necessary, place an eye shield over the eye patch. (See Chapter 3 for instructions on making a simple eye shield.) A light or semi-pressure patch should be applied to splint the eye only under certain conditions:

- Corneal abrasion requires a patch to allow the corneal epithelium to heal.
- Ocular surgery during which corneal epithelium or conjunctiva has been disrupted or damaged requires patching to put the eye at rest for healing.
- A patch is necessary after removal of a corneal foreign body (see below) provided that the corneal epithelium where the foreign body was embedded is not infected.

If an eye has been injured and infection is present, it should not be patched. When the eyelids are closed and covered with an eye pad, the surface of the eye becomes darker, warmer, and wetter, all conditions that promote bacterial infection.

Injuries to the eyelids

Contusion

Ecchymosis (blood in the subcutaneous tissue) causes the appearance of a 'black eye', which often results from contusion injury (blunt trauma). In contusion injury, the eyelids should be examined carefully for evidence of penetrating injury. A penetrating injury may not be evident because of swelling (edema) of the eyelids. The orbital rim (anterior orbital bone edges) should be palpated for evidence of fracture and displacement.

If no other ocular or adnexal injury is present, ecchymosis will clear more rapidly with warm compresses applied for 15 min every 6 hr. If the patient is examined and treated within a few min after injury, ice applied directly to the eyelids will help reduce swelling of the eyelids.

Laceration

An eyelid laceration is a surgical emergency. Primary repair of the laceration should be carried out as soon as possible after the injury has occurred. Penetrating injury of the eyeball should always be

Table 6 **Some causes of ocular injuries in developing nations**	
Household	Cultivating and harvesting crops; cutting and splitting firewood; burns from accidents at cooking fires (unattended children and epileptics may fall into cooking fires); insect sting or bite
Industrial	Often foreign bodies or penetrating ocular injuries (when required protective eye goggles or glasses are not worn); facial lacerations
Vehicle accidents	Broken glass from automobile windshields causes lacerations; seat belts can prevent facial injuries
Assault	Frequent facial lacerations, hyphema, and contusion injuries
Antipersonnel landmines	Traumatic amputation and perforating ocular injuries
Harmful eye practices	Traditional eye medications instilled into the eye; mechanical manipulation or thermal cautery by traditional healers

suspected when an eyelid laceration is present (**95**). Examination of the eyeball should be performed with great care if it is suspected that a corneal or scleral laceration is present. Because of ecchymosis, retraction of the eyelids with metal retractors may be necessary. (See Chapter 3 for instructions on making a simple eyelid retractor.)

Lacerations through the eyelid margin require special surgical attention. In addition to primary repair of each of the four layers of the eyelid, the eyelid margin should be carefully repaired. Care must be taken to remove all foreign bodies and dead (necrotic) tissue from the wound when repairing eyelid lacerations. Many eyelid injuries are contaminated with plant or vegetable foreign bodies.

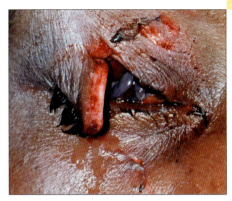

95 Full thickness upper eyelid laceration and lacerated globe from knife assault.

Lacrimal drainage system

A laceration through the eyelid and the lacrimal canaliculus should be repaired as soon after the injury as possible. Reattachment of the severed ends of the canaliculus is necessary to restore normal tear drainage. Be cautious in the surgical approach because the probe used in identifying the severed ends of the canaliculus may further damage the lacrimal drainage system if not handled carefully. A thin plastic and wire cannula may then be used to connect the severed ends. Thin plastic tubing may be left in place for several weeks to assist in anatomic healing of the canaliculus.

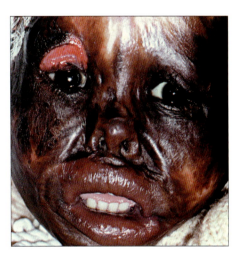

96 Facial burns and subsequent scarring from open cooking fire.

Burns

The blink reflex, a protective reflex, will usually cause the eyelids to close at the moment of burn injury, protecting the eyeball. Burns to the eyelids, even seemingly minor ones, may cause retraction of the eyelids and consequent exposure of the eyeball upon healing (**96**). The cornea must be protected during healing to prevent drying (exposure keratitis) and infection (corneal ulceration). Tarsorrhaphy (surgical closure of the upper and lower eyelids) should be carried out if the eyelids do not completely close or if skin and eyelid contracture begins to develop. Skin grafting of contracted eyelids from scarring is necessary for patients likely to develop exposure keratitis.

Immediate first aid for facial burns includes the following:

- Anesthesia medication to reduce pain.
- Washing and debridement of the burn site.
- Ice packs (if available) to reduce swelling.

Long-term management of burns includes:

- Systemic antibiotics (tetracycline or penicillin) orally in appropriate dosage (intramuscular antibiotics are not necessary if the patient is able to take oral medication).
- Protection of the burn area to prevent secondary infection.
- Regular debridement of necrotic tissue to encourage healing and prevent infection.

Orbital injuries

Injuries to the orbital structures may occur through contusion, eyelid laceration, or blunt injury to the eye or to its external supporting structures. Ocular movements in the six cardinal positions (see Chapter 15) may be affected. If double vision (diplopia) is present, there may be a fracture of the floor of the orbit. Strabismus may occur following orbital trauma.

After contusion injury, a careful examination is necessary to search for a possible penetrating wound to the orbit. A penetrating injury to the orbit usually requires surgical exploration and repair. Severe facial crush injuries, such as facial trauma sustained in automobile and industrial accidents, may also cause fractures of the orbital rim and/or the floor of the orbit. X-ray examination may be able to determine if a bony fracture is present. An 'air–fluid' level sign on X-ray in a maxillary sinus suggests orbital floor fracture.

Ocular surface injuries

Conjunctival injuries are usually minor but may obscure more serious injury to the sclera. Foreign bodies lodged in the conjunctiva are easily removed under topical anesthesia. Eyelid-infiltration anesthesia (local anesthetic) may be necessary before the eyelids can be retracted for an adequate examination. The eyelids must be everted (see Figure 166) to search for foreign material if a foreign body is suspected to be embedded in the tarsal conjunctiva. Removal of the foreign body may be carried out with small forceps. If there is a foreign body embedded in the conjunctiva, a penetrating or perforating injury to the sclera must be suspected.

Subconjunctival hemorrhage can occur from contusion injuries, even mild injuries, particularly in older patients, and from epidemic viral conjunctivitis. Elevated venous pressure, as encountered in sneezing and coughing, may cause subconjunctival hemorrhage. Warm compresses may reduce eyelid swelling and hasten absorption of the subconjunctival blood.

Swelling of the conjunctiva without hemorrhage (chemosis) often indicates an acute allergy. Such a reaction can also result from a foreign body that has lodged in the conjunctiva or in the eyelid fornices. Insects or insect parts lodged in the conjunctiva often cause a marked swelling reaction, and an insect sting or a spider bite should be suspected in a patient with acute eyelid swelling. Apply ice and administer an analgesic for pain. Any history of previous acute reactions should be determined in the case of insect sting reactions. Anaphylaxis – severe allergic reaction that can occur from insect stings, particularly bee stings – can result in death.

Lacerations of the conjunctiva should be debrided and thoroughly irrigated with sterile saline. Small, clean lacerations of a few millimeters will usually heal without surgical repair. More extensive lacerations of the conjunctiva require surgical repair under local anesthesia. Careful examination is necessary to look for a more serious scleral injury underneath the conjunctival laceration.

Corneal foreign body

Foreign bodies in the cornea are among the most common eye injuries (**97**); all are ocular emergencies and can result in severe and permanent damage if neglected. A variety of foreign substances are responsible: vegetable matter, such as chaff, maize, and leaf fragments in farmers; metal fragments in machinists; and wind-borne debris.

A patient with a corneal foreign body complains of pain, loss of vision, and tearing. Direct examination with the flashlight and magnifying glass or loupe will establish the diagnosis. The slit lamp is helpful but not essential to identify a corneal foreign body. Eyelid eversion may be necessary to identify a foreign body embedded in the tarsus of the upper eyelid that is causing corneal pain with blinking. Removal of the foreign body under topical anesthesia should be done immediately (**98**). If the foreign body cannot be removed with a cotton-tipped applicator, a 30-ga needle may be used to lift out the object. The bevel of the needle should be facing up and the cornea should be approached from the temporal side. Small metallic foreign bodies can be removed by twirling a cotton-tipped applicator over the foreign body. If the foreign body is deeply

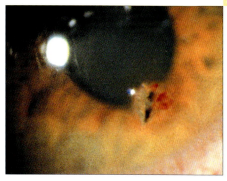

97 Embedded corneal foreign body.

embedded in the cornea, surgical removal under peribulbar block may be necessary. The corneal epithelial defect produced by a foreign body should be managed as a corneal abrasion. Instill an antibiotic ointment without corticosteroid in the inferior fornix and apply an occlusive eye patch. Examine the cornea 24 hours later; fluorescein dye will confirm epithelial healing or lack of it. A persistent abrasion from a foreign body can result in a corneal ulcer (see Chapter 11 , External disease, for treatment of corneal ulcer). Fungal corneal ulcer should be suspected as a late complication of non-healing corneal abrasion due to a vegetable (plant matter) corneal foreign body.

98 Removal of a corneal foreign body. Remove foreign body with cotton-tipped applicator (a). If foreign body cannot be removed with cotton-tipped applicator, attempt removal with 30-ga needle, bevel up (b).

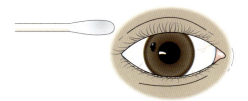

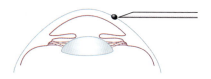

a

b

Corneal abrasion

Corneal abrasion – a scratch in the corneal epithelium – is a common ocular injury. A corneal abrasion may result from a seemingly small or trivial injury. Pain, tearing, and loss of vision are symptoms. The diagnosis is made by staining the cornea with fluorescein dye. The corneal epithelial defect will appear bright green, whereas the normal corneal epithelium will not stain. Treatment is the same as for corneal abrasion due to a small corneal foreign body as described above.

A drop of topical anesthetic will provide instant relief from the pain resulting from a corneal foreign body or corneal abrasion. *Topical ocular anesthetics must never be given to patients for outpatient use. Serious and permanent corneal damage can result from overuse of these anesthetics.*

A 'corneal burn' can result from exposure to the arc light used in metal welding. This can be prevented if the welder wears appropriate protective eyewear. A patient with a welder's arc burn complains of pain, loss of vision, and tearing. Fluorescein dye reveals widespread corneal punctate (dot) staining, usually in both eyes. Management is the same as for corneal abrasion. Sunlamp keratitis and snow blindness (corneal injuries not commonly seen in tropical countries!) are also managed as corneal abrasions.

Corneal chemical injuries

Chemical injuries of the cornea require immediate first aid and prompt follow-up treatment. If gasoline (petrol), an industrial chemical, or any other chemical substance has been splashed into the eyes, the immediate first aid treatment is irrigation (lavage) of the involved eye with clean water. If a water tap is available, the patient's head should be positioned under running water, the eyelids retracted, and both eyes lavaged for at least 5 minutes. Examination should be carried out after lavage with tap water (or with sterile saline if available). Use a drop of topical anesthetic if the patient cannot open the eyes without pain. Also examine the bulbar and tarsal conjunctiva (with eyelid eversion) and the cornea for foreign bodies that may have been splashed into the eye(s) with the chemical.

Alkaline (basic) substances – chemicals with a pH greater than 7.0 – are highly damaging to the cornea. Examples include lye (NaOH, or sodium hydroxide compounds), cleaning fluids, and calcium hydroxide (used in building materials). These chemicals can penetrate the cornea in seconds or minutes. Immediate and copious lavage with tap water or sterile saline is the best hope of preserving a clear and healthy cornea. Lavage should continue until the pH becomes neutral. The pH may be tested with litmus paper or urine test strips.

Corneal abrasion may result from chemical injury. Confirm the diagnosis of corneal abrasion with fluorescein dye, as described above.

Good safety practices in handling chemicals will prevent eye injuries. Industrial safety for factory workers should be promoted at the workplace to prevent low vision and blindness.

Contusion to the eyeball

Severe contusion usually causes injury to intraocular structures that often results in permanent low vision or blindness. Significant intraocular effects include hyphema, iridoplegia, lens dislocation, and fundus injury.

Hyphema
Hyphema, or blood in the anterior chamber, can result from a direct blow to the eye. Blood settles out into a layer in the inferior anterior chamber when the patient is standing (**99**). Conservative management of recent hyphema is as follows:

- Bed rest for 3 days with sedation, if necessary.
- Bilateral patching (to rest both eyes).
- Do not use miotic drops.

Hyphema can recur even during hospitalization, particularly if the patient is not at complete rest. Rebleeding most often occurs on the third day after the initial injury. Total hyphema ('black-ball' hyphema) fills the anterior chamber with blood, blocks aqueous drainage, and produces high intraocular pressure and blood staining of the corneal endothelium.

Surgical removal of the clotted blood in the anterior chamber is necessary. Secondary glaucoma can be a late complication of hyphema, even from a small hyphema. Damage to the trabecular drainage tissue in the angle and tearing (ripping) of the iris at the iris base attachment to the ciliary body can occur from a contusion injury that causes hyphema. This condition is called *angle recession*. All hyphema patients should be reexamined regularly because of their risk of developing secondary glaucoma.

Iridoplegia
Contusion injury to the iris can cause loss of normal iris function as a result of damage to the iris muscles. Traumatic mydriasis (traumatic iridoplegia) is a pupil that is chronically dilated due to ocular injury. Such a pupil is unreactive to light and usually unresponsive to mydriatics and miotics. The condition is often permanent.

Lens dislocation
Severe contusion to the eyeball may dislocate (luxate) or partially dislocate (subluxate) the lens (**100**). The lens may be dislocated posteriorly into the vitreous or anteriorly into the anterior chamber.

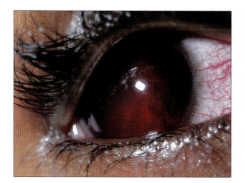

99 Nearly total hyphema (blood in the anterior chamber) resulting from contusion injury.

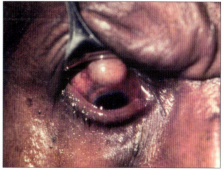

100 Ethiopian cattle herder with subconjunctival lens caused by contusion injury; the lens entered the subconjunctival space through scleral rupture.

A lens dislocated into the anterior chamber often blocks outflow of aqueous and produces acute high intraocular pressure. Corneal edema will complicate excessively high intraocular pressure. Tearing (ripping) of the iris, hyphema, and vitreous bleeding may accompany lens dislocation. Immediate surgical removal of a lens dislocated into the anterior chamber is necessary to save the eye. Partial dislocation of the lens may cause angle recession and secondary glaucoma.

Ocular fundus injuries

Severe contusion injuries can result in serious damage to the ocular fundus. If the red fundus reflex normally seen with direct ophthalmoscopy is obscured after a contusion injury, blood may be present in the vitreous.

Retinal detachment (separation of the retina from its attachment to the sclera) may result from contusion injury. Retinal detachment should be suspected in a patient with vitreous hemorrhage. A tear in the retina across a blood vessel will produce vitreous hemorrhage and a dark or black fundus reflex. Patients with vitreous hemorrhage should be examined regularly. Retinal detachment, if present, cannot be surgically repaired until the blood has cleared out of the vitreous.

Contusion injuries can produce macular edema, which will reduce visual acuity. The macular area appears raised and wrinkled when edema is present. Optic atrophy may also result from ocular contusion injuries.

Penetrating injuries to the eyeball

Penetrating injuries to the eyeball often result in severe damage to intraocular structures. *A penetrating injury to the eyeball is a serious surgical emergency. Appropriate treatment must be instituted immediately.*

Deeply embedded corneal foreign bodies that have penetrated the cornea or sclera should be removed in the operating room under sterile conditions. Corneal and scleral lacerations with or without iris or iris/ciliary body prolapse should be operated on immediately after the diagnosis has been established (**101**, **102**, **103**).

Prolapsed uveal tissue (iris, ciliary body, and choroid) should be excised and the scleral and corneal wounds repaired with 9-0 or 10-0 nylon suture. Prolapsed and exposed uvea can cause a severe granulomatous uveitis in the remaining normal eye, a condition known as *sympathetic ophthalmia*. This serious late complication can result in the loss of the normal eye.

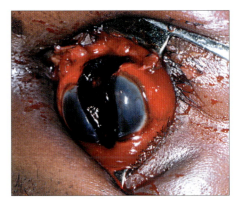

101 Corneal laceration extending into the lens and ciliary body.

Great care should be taken to remove all prolapsed uveal tissue at the time of surgical repair. If the lens has been perforated by the injury, it should be removed, along with all loose lens fragments.

Injectable subconjunctival corticosteroids, frequent topical corticosteroids, and topical atropine 1% are used in postoperative management of these severe injuries. A booster intramuscular dose of 0.5 cc of tetanus toxoid (for a patient previously immunized) should be administered. Tetanus hyperimmune sera may be necessary for patients with open and contaminated injuries to the adnexa and eyeball.

A *ruptured globe* refers to an eyeball with an extensive corneoscleral injury. Useful vision in many of these severely injured eyes is difficult to salvage even under the best of surgical circumstances. A severely inflamed and sightless eye after surgical repair of a corneal or scleral laceration should be enucleated or eviscerated. This will reduce the risk of sympathetic ophthalmia.

Intraocular foreign bodies

A variety of substances and small particles may enter the eye in severe penetrating injury. All are serious ocular injuries and should be removed under sterile conditions in the operating room promptly after the diagnosis has been established.

Metallic intraocular foreign body injuries commonly occur in the industrial workplace, and the diagnosis can easily be missed. A history of sudden and painless loss of vision in a worker hammering on metal is classic. A tiny entrance wound through conjunctiva and sclera may be missed during the ocular examination. Frontal and lateral X-rays will assist in making the diagnosis if the intraocular foreign body is metallic, although X-ray examination may not reveal a very small metallic intraocular foreign body. If the particle is located in the posterior segment, indirect ophthalmoscopy will be required to visualize it. If the foreign body has perforated the lens, causing a secondary cataract, it may not be visible even with indirect ophthalmoscopy.

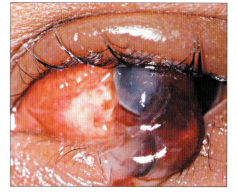

102 Ruptured globe with iris and ciliary body prolapse.

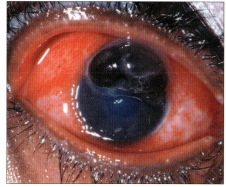

103 Iris prolapse from corneal perforation.

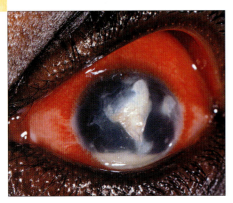

104 Intracorneal vegetable matter with hypopyon.

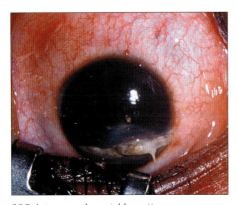

105 Intracorneal vegetable matter.

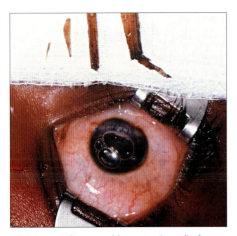

106 Intraocular vegetable matter (wood) after removal and repair.

Once the object is identified, extraction of a metallic foreign body is performed under sterile operating room conditions with an electromagnet or under direct visualization under microscopy.

Intraocular foreign body injuries involving vegetable matter often result in bacterial or fungal endophthalmitis and subsequent loss of the eye. Intraocular vegetable matter (wood splinters, for example) must be surgically removed as soon as possible if the injured eye is to be saved (**104–106**).

Radiographic scanning instruments – computerized tomography (CT) and magnetic resonance imaging (MRI) – may be available only in the best-equipped tertiary centers. These instruments are valuable for detecting and locating intraocular foreign bodies.

Harmful eye practices

Traditional healers may use mechanical manipulation or thermal cautery on the ocular adnexa or may instill medications onto the surface of the eye(s) that can cause harm. Traditional eye medication (TEM) may include extracts from leaves or herbs, human urine, or animal products, and often causes permanent damage to the ocular surface, visual impairment, and blindness. Plant substances that are chemically basic (pH greater than 7.0) can be particularly harmful because they may penetrate the cornea and cause permanent

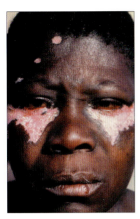

107 Thermal cautery causing scarring by traditional healer; intended to treat trachoma; note lower lid ectropion caused by the thermal cautery.

opacity or perforate the cornea and cause endophthalmitis. Traditional healers may also use thermal cautery to treat eyelid lesions, infection, and entropion (**107**). Such treatments that cause damage to the ocular adnexa, to the eye, and to vision are collectively known as harmful eye practices (HEP).

Because traditional healers are respected in villages and rural communities, they should not be stigmatized by allopathic health care practitioners. Rather, they can be trained to avoid certain practices that are harmful to the eyes and instead to utilize treatments that are known to be beneficial. Several projects in Africa include traditional healers in their health care delivery systems. By doing so, harmful eye practices may be avoided or lessened.

Antipersonnel landmines

The antipersonnel landmine (APL), a passive instrument of war, has become a major global public health problem. Armed APLs may be detonated by the pressure of a footfall long after they have been placed in the ground for military purposes. More civilians than soldiers are maimed, blinded, or killed by APLs.

Approximately 80–100 million APLs have been left in the earth in more than 66 countries, most of them in the developing world. Countries of southeast Asia, the Middle East, southern Africa, and Central America are the most severely affected. Cambodia, with a population of approximately 10 million people, has an estimated 10 million APLs in its soil. Egypt, Afghanistan, and Mozambique are also heavily mined with APLs.

Children are particularly at risk of injury from APLs because they may handle the mines when they find them lying on the ground (**108**). There are more than 20,000 deaths and injuries from APLs every year. Ninety percent of all APL injuries are to civilians.

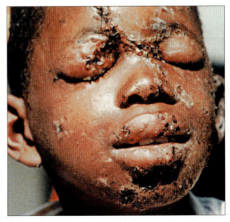

108 Mozambican boy with facial and eye injuries from an antipersonnel landmine explosion.

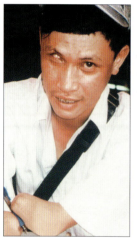

109 Mozambican war injury (shrapnel) and endophthalmitis.

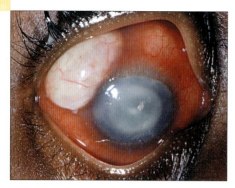

110 Vietnamese man who lost one leg, both forearms, and one eye to an antipersonnel landmine.

Mutilation and blindness result in those victims who survive APL blasts (**109**, **110**). Recent data from two Cambodia surveys indicate that APL explosions are a significant cause of both monocular and binocular blindness in the civilian population, much larger than previously assumed (**111**, **112**).

The International Campaign to Ban Landmines has secured a treaty to ban the manufacture, use, and transfer of APLs. The treaty was signed by representatives of 121 nations in Ottawa, Canada, in December 1997. The legacy of currently armed APLs will remain with us for many years. The international campaign seeks to do the following:

- Ban manufacture of all APLs.
- Ban all future use of APLs.
- Destroy all stockpiles of APLs.
- End international trade in APLs.
- Rehabilitate APL survivors.

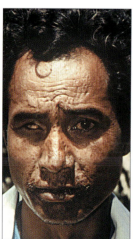

111 Cambodian man who survived smallpox but lost an eye to an antipersonnel landmine explosion.

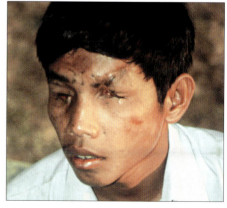

112 Cambodian man who lost an arm and an eye to a landmine explosion.

9

Onchocerciasis

An ounce of prevention is worth a pound of cure.
Proverb

Onchocerciasis ('river blindness') is a chronic parasitic infection that can cause corneal and retinal scarring and intraocular damage from uveitis. Approximately 18 million people are infected with the disease in 30 African and six Latin American countries; the great majority of the 270,000 people blind from onchocerciasis are in Africa. Approximately 110 million people are at risk of contracting the disease. Blindness from onchocerciasis is preventable by controlling the infection itself with systemic ivermectin and by effective management of the early stages of resultant keratitis, chorioretinitis, and uveitis.

Natural history

Onchocerciasis is caused by a parasitic nematode worm, *Onchocerca volvulus* (113), which is transmitted by the bite of a blackfly of the genus *Simulium* (114). *Simulium damnosum* is the species most frequently implicated in the transmission of the *Onchocerca volvulus* microfilariae (larvae) in African endemic areas. Onchocerciasis is known as 'river blindness' because the disease occurs near fast-flowing rivers where the blackfly breeds.

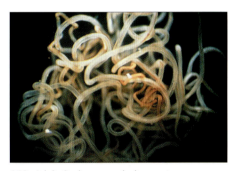

113 Adult *Onchocerca volvulus*.

A female blackfly must feed on blood in order to ovulate. When she bites an infected human host she ingests the microscopic microfilariae that are present in the skin. These develop over 2–3 weeks inside the fly to become larger, infective-stage larvae, which are then are transmitted to another human host when she bites. The infectious larvae develop into adult worms, forming nodules beneath the skin.

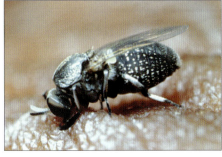

114 Biting *Simulium* blackfly.

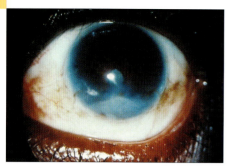

115 Advanced inflammatory reaction in the cornea and iris caused by microfilaria in the eye.

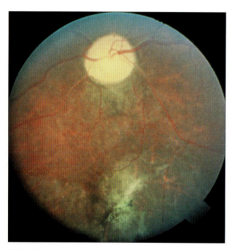

116 Optic atrophy and retinal scarring, secondary to onchocerciasis.

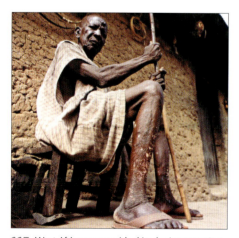

117 West African man with skin depigmentation and adult *Onchocerca volvulus* nodules.

These skin nodules are a few millimeters to a centimeter thick, often forming on bony prominences such as the head, shoulder blades, and hips. Adult female worms in the nodules can be up to 1 m long and are coiled up like a ball of string; they can, over their lifespan of 15 years, produce millions of microfilariae. Male worms travel between the nodules to inseminate the females. The microfilariae migrate throughout the body and can be found in the bloodstream and in some internal organs. They are found in high concentration in the skin and eye.

Pathways to blindness from onchocerciasis

Corneal scarring, chorioretinitis and chorioretinal scarring, and optic atrophy from microfilarial invasion of the eye are the major pathways to blindness in onchocerciasis (**115, 116**). Uveitis (inflammation of a part or all of the uveal tract) may occur when microfilariae penetrate the sclera and enter the eyeball. Onchocerciasis can also result in low vision or permanent blindness by causing secondary cataract and secondary glaucoma.

Diagnosis

Patients with active onchocerciasis with ocular involvement complain of eye pain and loss of vision. The diagnosis can be confirmed by skin snip and examination of the specimen for microfilariae under the microscope. Common clinical signs of systemic onchocerciasis are skin nodules and patchy loss of skin pigment (**117**), along with skin rash and itching.

In patients with severe infection, microfilariae may be seen in the cornea and anterior chamber with the slit lamp. Dead microfilarie in the cornea appear as straight, transparent needles, whereas living microfilariae are coiled up, and usually seen in the peripheral cornea, particularly at 3 and 9 o'clock positions (×25 magnification required). To easily see swimming microfilariae in the anterior chamber, the patient should keep the head down for 2 minutes before examination with the slit lamp (×10 magnification sufficient). There is often a chronic 'torpid' iritis in these cases, and the beam of the slit lamp will show in the anterior chamber (flare) and cells can be seen under high magnification. Iritis may be present with corneal infiltration.

Punctate keratitis with snowflake-like stromal opacities may occur with corneal microfilarial lesions. A whitish patch in the cornea, initially as a limbal infiltrate at 3 and 9 o'clock, indicates deep corneal scarring (sclerosing keratitis) which may be progressive, semilunate, and blinding.

Indirect ophthalmoscopy will be required to fully visualize chorioretinal changes, which usually occur in the posterior pole and midperiphery. Inactive chorioretinitis from onchocerciasis – a black or darkly pigmented scar with large whitish patches – may be seen with careful ophthalmoscopy. In advanced cases there is often also optic nerve disease (atrophy) present.

Management

Medical management
Systemic treatment of onchocerciasis can control generalized onchocercal infection. Treatment cannot reverse permanent visual disability or blindness from the disease but often halts further progression. In the past, diethylcarbamazine citrate (DEC) and suramin sodium were used to control systemic onchocerciasis, but they have been replaced by ivermectin (Mectizan), a broad-spectrum antiparasitic drug (**118**). Ivermectin is a much safer drug for human use than DEC and suramin

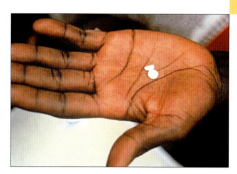

118 Ivermectin (Mectizan) dose.

sodium, which are now considered dangerous for the treatment of onchocerciasis because of serious side effects.

Ivermectin acts by killing microfilariae in infected patients. Thus, the progression of onchocercal eye infections that produce blindness can be prevented. Ivermectin can also reduce or stop dermatitis and itching caused by microfilariae and can prevent progression of disfiguring skin changes caused by onchocerciasis. Ivermectin also suppresses the release of viable microfilariae by the adult female worm.

By reducing the microfilariae population with ivermectin treatment of individual patients and of communities, there is less chance for the microfilariae to be transmitted by the *Simulium* blackfly vector. In this way, transmission of the disease can be reduced by means of large-scale treatment with ivermectin.

Ivermectin does not kill the adult *Onchocerca* worms nor does it reverse blindness or advanced skin changes due to scarring. Infective larvae introduced into humans by the blackfly are not killed by the drug and can still develop into adult worms.

Minor side effects associated with ivermectin may include headache, skin rash, itching, muscle pain, and fever. These conditions usually settle quickly with aspirin or acetaminophen.

The following patient groups should not receive ivermectin:

- Children, either younger than 5 years of age, or weighing less than 15 kg, or less than 90 cm in height (**119**).
- Pregnant women.
- Women breastfeeding children who are younger than 1 week of age.
- Persons with meningitis or other serious acute or chronic illness.

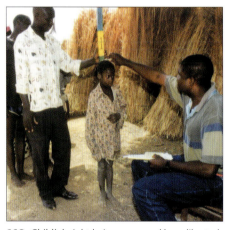

119 Child's height being measured by calibrated stick to determine Mectizan® dosage.

Table 7 **Ivermectin dosage**

Body weight (kg)	Height (cm)	Annual dose (mg)
<15	<90	do not give
15–24	90–119	3
25–44	120–140	6
45–64	141–158	9
>64	>158	12

The correct dosage of ivermectin, given once per year, is determined by either weight or height (*Table 7*). Originally distributed as 6-mg tablets, ivermectin is now available as 3-mg tablets; this simplifies dosage. Patients should be observed by treatment staff as they receive and swallow the correct number of tablets.

Management of ocular onchocerciasis

Management of patients with ocular onchocerciasis is directed toward control of keratitis, chorioretinitis, secondary complications, and, occasionally, anterior uveitis. (See Chapter 12 for more detailed discussion of the management of uveitis.) While cure of ocular complications from onchocerciasis is not possible, vision may be preserved and improved with good management of ocular complications secondary to the disease. Onchocerciasis uveitis and its sequelae make filtering surgery for glaucoma and cataract surgery risky, but such surgery can be performed provided that the uveitis is controlled at the time of surgery. Eyes with severe uveitis from onchocerciasis and other causes may develop phthisis bulbi after intraocular surgery. The prognosis in corneal grafting for onchocercal scarring is poor because patients frequently have extensive and blinding chorioretinitis. Cataract surgery in a patient with corneal damage may not be beneficial.

Surgical management

Nodulectomy (surgical removal of large nodules of adult worms, larvae, and microfilariae) from the skin may reduce the parasite load somewhat but does not necessarily improve or prevent eye complications. Many nodules are deeply buried in the skin and subcutaneous tissue and cannot be surgically excised. In most cases nodulectomy is not warranted.

Elimination of onchocerciasis blindness

The strategy for reducing ocular morbidity, visual disability, and blindness from onchocerciasis is twofold:

- To reduce microfilarial loads in infected individuals and in communities in endemic areas by use of ivermectin.
- To interrupt the transmission of the disease by controlling the *Simulium* blackfly vector.

Merck & Co., Inc. (which operates as Merck, Sharp & Dohme in many countries outside of the United States) provides iver-mectin (Mectizan) free of charge to all endemic countries for the elimination of onchocerciasis, through the Mectizan Donation Program (MDP). Ministries of Health and any interested collaborative organization can apply for Mectizan for large-scale public health use. The World Bank has provided major funding for iver-mectin distribution since the Mectizan Donation Program began in 1988 through the Onchocerciasis Control Program in West Africa (OCP, 1974–2002), and currently through the African Programme for Onchocerciasis Control (APOC), which is managed by WHO as the coordinating body for ivermectin distribution in the African region. In Latin America, the Onchocerciasis Elimination Program of the Americas (OEPA) is successfully pursuing the ultimate elimination of the disease from the Western Hemisphere; current progress indicates that there should be no more eye lesions from onchocerciasis after 2007 in the six countries concerned.

Non-governmental organizations working in areas where onchocerciasis is endemic collaborate with national min-istries of health to distribute the medica-tion to those infected or at risk of infection. Distribution of ivermectin was initially usually conducted in communities by rural health care teams, but a community-directed treatment scheme is being suc-cessfully implemented in the APOC countries, covering at present approxi-mately 45 million people annually. It is carefully supervised to ensure appropriate surveillance and reporting of any adverse reactions to treatment, particularly in areas co-endemic for Loiasis, another filarial disease known to (rarely) provoke serious adverse experiences in highly infested patients being treated with Mectizan. Caution must therefore be exercised when treating an onchocerciasis patient, who may also have a high load of Loa loa.

The WHO implemented a long-term blackfly control program in West Africa from 1974 (OCP, see above). It aimed to reduce transmission of onchocerciasis by controlling the *Simulium* vector by aerial spraying of environmentally friendly insec-ticides (**120**). The aerial spraying program was one of the largest public health projects ever undertaken, but it encoun-tered problems with insecticide resistance, and therefore switched much of its opera-tions to large-scale Mectizan distribution since 1988. The OCP closed down in 2002, having successfully controlled onchocer-ciasis in most of the 11 West African countries in the OCP region.

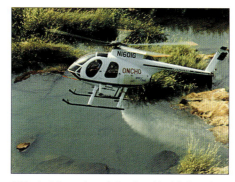

120 Aerial spraying of *Simulium* blackfly breeding site in West Africa.

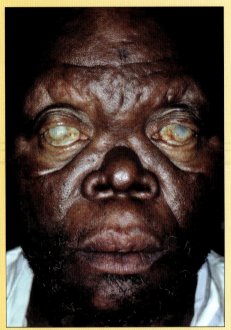

The face of leprosy: corneal scarring, loss of eyelid lashes and brow hair, and sunken bridge of nose.

10

Leprosy

Leprosy patients form a severely disadvantaged group because of other disabilities due to the disease, its social stigma, and the difficulties and delay in receiving appropriate eye care.
Paul Courtright

People need not go blind from leprosy. For the primary prevention of blindness, early detection and systemic treatment of leprosy are of utmost importance.
Gordon F. Johnson

Leprosy, also known as Hansen's disease, is a chronic, slowly developing, debilitating disease that affects skin, peripheral nerves, and extremities. When it involves skin and nerves of the face, it may cause lepromata (lesions), facial nerve palsy, lagophthalmos, loss of eyelashes, exposure keratitis, corneal opacity, uveitis, and secondary glaucoma. Low vision or blindness may result.

Ocular complications from leprosy and resulting visual impairment and blindness can be prevented by early detection and treatment. All eye health care workers who live in regions of the world where leprosy occurs should be trained in recognition and treatment of ocular leprosy.

Leprosy is caused by the bacterium *Mycobacterium leprae*. Multibacillary leprosy patients are those who have a minimal immune response to the leprosy bacillus. These patients accumulate millions of leprosy bacilli in their tissues. Advanced cases have a typical leonine ('lion-like') facial appearance. Paucibacillary leprosy patients have a greater immune response to the bacilli and therefore accumulate far fewer bacilli in their tissues.

The immune response itself may be very damaging to tissues despite the small number of bacilli. Corneal opacity, limbal lepromata and adnexal lepromata, chronic uveitis, lagophthalmos, and cataract are typical of multibacillary disease, while paucibacillary disease typically may result in lagophthalmos and cataract without the more pronounced multibacillary lesions. Leprosy uveitis tends to be quiet and low grade, and results in miotic pupils with posterior synechiae and secondary cataract. Multibacillary has replaced the term 'lepromatous,' and paucibacillary has replaced the term 'tuberculoid.'

Epidemiology

Leprosy has become stigmatized during its long history as a disease known to cause disfiguring lesions of the face and loss of fingers and toes. Leprosy patients often are isolated from families, households, and communities because of their appearance and fear of others contracting the disease.

Transmission of the disease appears to involve long exposure to those who are infected with the leprosy bacterium. It is apparently not transmitted by only a few contacts with affected individuals but by longstanding contact, such as in families.

Regions where leprosy is more concentrated are sub-Saharan Africa, the Middle East, the Indian subcontinent, Indochina, and islands of the western Pacific. Although a disease largely associated with tropical regions, leprosy also occurs in temperate countries such as Korea, Mexico, and Argentina, and may in fact occur in any climate. For example, it was formerly common in Norway (where it was described by Hansen in 1873, hence the alternative name Hansen's disease). It is commonly associated with poverty and disappears when socioeconomic conditions improve.

According to the World Health Organization, between 1985 and 2005, more than 14 million leprosy patients completed multi-drug treatment (MDT) (see page 148). In 2004, approximately 460,000 patients were registered for treatment worldwide. There are no reliable data on the number of leprosy patients with low vision and blindness due to their disease, although it is believed that as many as one-third of all patients suffer from disabilities, including loss of digits; numbness (anesthesia) of extremities, skin, and face; lesions of the extremities and face; and visual impairment often leading to blindness.

Pathways to blindness from leprosy

Corneal opacity

Mycobacterium leprae can invade the cornea and cause opacities (maculae or nebulae). The bacteria invade the cornea along the pathways of the corneal nerves. Corneal sensitivity is often lost, and the cornea may become anesthetic.

Punctate corneal lesions (punctate keratitis) in the epithelium are common with ocular leprosy complications. Without pain sensation, corneal injuries are not noticed by the patient. In an anesthetic cornea, even small corneal foreign bodies and abrasions can result in severe corneal erosion, ulceration, and scarring.

Leprosy may cause paralysis of the seventh cranial (facial) nerve, resulting in failure of proper eyelid function. The upper eyelid fails to close properly (lagophthalmos); the lower eyelid may be lax and droop. With failure of normal eyelid closure, the cornea is continuously exposed and becomes dry due to lack of the tear film that is normally provided by normal eyelid function (exposure keratitis). Bacterial infection or corneal ulceration with corneal perforation and endophthalmitis or corneal scarring is usually the result.

Surgically suturing the eyelids together (tarsorrhaphy) will prevent exposure keratitis. The tarsorrhaphy may be left in place until the seventh nerve recovers its normal function, although it seldom does in lepromatous nerve palsy. If seventh nerve function recovers, the tarsorrhaphy may be removed. If a permanent tarsorrhaphy is required, a small opening between the sutured eyelids should be maintained to provide a pinhole opening for vision.

Uveitis

All leprosy patients with ocular complaints should be carefully examined for evidence of anterior uveitis (iridocyclitis). Posterior uveitis (chorioretinitis) is rarely caused by leprosy; if posterior uveitis is present, other causes must be suspected. Signs and symptoms of uveitis from leprosy are the same as for tuberculosis and include hazy cornea, cells and flare in the anterior chamber, and failure of the pupil to constrict normally to light. (See Chapter 12 for signs, symptoms, and management of uveitis.)

If not treated accurately and promptly, permanent intraocular damage may result. The iris may adhere to the anterior lens capsule (posterior synechiae; see Figure 74). If the entire pupillary border adheres to the lens, aqueous is prevented from entering the anterior chamber through the pupil. The iris then bulges forward, a condition known as iris bombé (see Figure 75). If the iris adheres to the peripheral cornea, peripheral anterior synechiae may result, which block the outflow of aqueous fluid by obstructing the trabecular meshwork (see Figure 76). Both posterior synechiae and peripheral anterior synechiae contribute to glaucoma which, if not diagnosed and treated, may result in blindness or severe loss of vision.

Cataract

Secondary cataract from uveitis and glaucoma (complicated cataract) may occur in leprosy patients. Age-related cataract may already be present. Patients with existing cataract may experience worsening cataract upon contraction of leprosy. Uveitis and glaucoma due to leprosy may cause the cataract to become more dense or opaque.

Diagnosis

Health care workers working at the primary level in countries and regions where leprosy is known to occur should be trained to recognize systemic signs of leprosy. All eye care workers – ophthalmic assistants, clinical officers, nurses, and ophthalmologists – should be able to recognize the typical ocular signs of leprosy and should be able to diagnose the disease.

Typical systemic signs may include the following:
- Loss or absorption of fingers and toes.
- Loss of sensation in hands, forearms, feet, and lower legs.
- Chronic ulcers of the extremities that do not heal.
- Nodules (lepromata) of the extremities or trunk.

Typical ocular signs may include the following:
- Complaints of eye pain and decreased vision.
- Chronic conjunctivitis or discharge from the eye.
- Drooping lower eyelids; failure of eyelids to close properly (**121**).

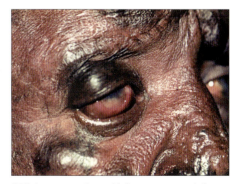

121 Leprosy patient with lepromata, ptosis from facial nerve palsy, and loss of eyelashes and eyebrows.

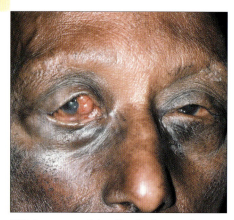

122 Lepromata of the ciliary body extending to the sclera and cornea.

- Corneal clouding, ulceration, or scarring.
- Lepromata of the ocular adnexa, the ciliary body, or on the corneoscleral surface (**122**).
- Signs of uveitis such as cells and flare in the anterior chamber (visible with the slit lamp).
- Failure of the pupil to constrict normally to light.

Treatment

The chronic nature of leprosy and the lack of definite scientific knowledge of how it is transmitted make it a difficult disease to prevent and treat. There is no vaccine available for people at high risk of contracting the disease. Medical treatment is long term. Surgery is performed after leprosy has already caused physical deformity or dysfunction.

Medical

Recommended treatment for leprosy is now multidrug therapy (MDT) with one regime for multibacillary patients and one for paucibacillary patients, as follows:

Multibacillary patients

(to be given for at least 1 year)
1   Rifampicin: 600 mg once monthly, supervised.
2   Clofazimine: 300 mg once monthly, supervised; and 50 mg daily, self-administered.
3   Dapsone: 100 mg daily, self-administered.

Paucibacillary patients

(to be given for 6 months)
1   Rifampicin: 600 mg once monthly, supervised.
2   Dapsone: 100 mg daily, self-administered.

Rifampicin and dapsone must be adjusted for low body weight (<35 kg).

If leprosy is diagnosed by the ophthalmic health care worker, the ocular lesions should not be treated without attention to the systemic disease. Medical treatment of the disease should be carried out by the leprosy control officer at the same time that ocular complications of leprosy are being treated by the eye health care worker. The eye health care worker is only one

member of the leprosy treatment and rehabilitation team, and systemic treatment of
leprosy must be a component of the eye
care treatment program.

Surgical

Ocular surgical services for leprosy
patients may include any of the following:

- Protection of the cornea by partial
  eyelid closure (tarsorrhaphy) if
  indicated by corneal exposure from
  lagophthalmos.
- Plastic repair of lower eyelid ectropion.
- Peripheral iridectomy for glaucoma
  secondary to iris bombé.
- Filtering surgery (trabeculectomy or
  thermal sclerostomy) for primary
  glaucoma or glaucoma secondary to
  intraocular leprosy complications.
- Excision of lepromata from the eye or
  ocular adnexa if the lepromata cause
  dysfunction or impairment of vision.
- Cataract surgery for age-related or
  complicated cataract. Cataract surgery
  in leprosy patients can be difficult and
  must be carefully considered. In
  addition to technical difficulty in
  extracting the lens without intraoperative complications, ocular hypertension
  and uveitis may occur and worsen the
  postoperative course. Potential benefits
  of better visual acuity and peripheral
  vision must be weighed against
  possible severe surgical complications.

Other non-ocular surgical services for
rehabilitation of leprosy patients include
reconstruction of limb deformities, tendon
release surgery for contractures of fingers
and toes, skin grafting (especially for burns
sustained because of nerve and skin anesthesia), and debridement of skin and limb
ulcers.

Leprosy and public health

A comprehensive national leprosy program
is necessary for control of the disease,
requiring the support of senior health care
administrators. Leprosy patients should be
registered for treatment with the national
or regional control program. Patients with
advanced leprosy and complications may
be hospitalized at a long-term facility for
treatment, reconstructive surgery, and
rehabilitation. For example, the All-Africa
Leprosy Rehabilitation and Training
(ALERT) Center in Addis Ababa, Ethiopia, is
a leprosy program resource center for
Africa. Patients are treated and rehabilitat-
ed there, and health care workers are
trained in all aspects of caring for leprosy
patients.

Leprosy patients may be registered for
treatment at home if they live in a country
or region with a leprosy control program
that includes village visitation by rural
health care workers. Primary or rural
health care workers visit patients in their
communities for diagnosis, treatment, and
referral if necessary. A model community
control program for leprosy is maintained
in Malawi. Primary health care workers on
bicycles or motorbikes are able to reach
rural areas in Malawi for regular treatment
of leprosy patients who do not have complications requiring hospitalization.

Social aspects of leprosy

The terms 'leper' and 'leper colony' have
come to acquire negative meanings and
should not be used by anyone working
with the treatment and rehabilitation of
those with the disease. 'Hansen's disease'
or 'leprosy patient' are terms that are not
stigmatized and should be used instead
when referring to people who have contracted leprosy. The dignity of all patients
must be recognized, respected, and
protected by all health care workers.

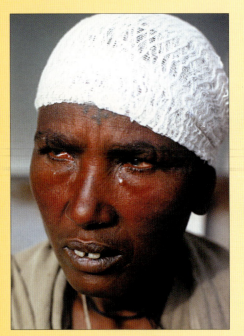

Ethiopian woman with bilateral bacterial conjunctivitis.

11

External disease

Mine eyes are full of tears, I cannot see.
Shakespeare, *Richard II*

External ocular disease is a major cause of blindness and low vision in the developing world. Certain external disease problems may also cause only ocular irritation, but certain potentially serious external ocular surface conditions may begin with minimal symptoms. Trachoma (Chapter 7) and corneal complications of malnutrition (Chapter 4) are significant subjects in themselves and are discussed separately. This chapter presents other significant external ocular, adnexal and surface diseases.

Conjunctivitis

Conjunctivitis is a general description, often used imprecisely, that covers numerous different types and causes of conjunctivitis. 'Conjunctivitis' is one of the most common ocular diagnoses recorded for patients presenting to rural outpatient clinics in many developing nations. An accurate diagnosis for each patient with conjunctivitis must be made before appropriate treatment can be instituted. Antibiotics are often given to patients for conjunctivitis when treatment is not necessary. (Refer to Appendix A for a comparative description of conjunctivitis and other causes of red eye.)

Non-purulent conjunctivitis

Non-purulent conjunctivitis is characterized by pinkish or reddish conjunctiva.

Viral conjunctivitis

Viral conjunctivitis is caused by one of a variety of viruses that infect the bulbar and tarsal conjunctiva. The typical characteristics of viral conjunctivitis are as follows:

- Visual acuity usually is not affected.
- It is usually bilateral.
- The conjunctiva is diffusely red from vascular reaction.
- Enlarged preauricular lymph nodes may be present.
- Follicles may be present in the conjunctiva, especially the upper eyelid tarsal conjunctiva.
- Serous (fluid) discharge may be present.

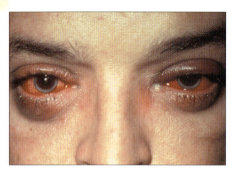

123 Bilateral epidemic viral conjunctivitis.

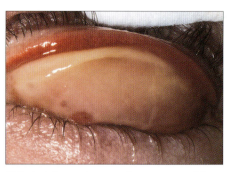

124 An inflammatory membrane may result from severe inflammatory viral conjunctivitis.

The infection can be spread by respiratory droplets from an infected patient to other people by coughing and sneezing. Epidemic viral conjunctivitis is seasonal and is common when 'colds' and viral upper respiratory infections are prevalent or epidemic.

Staining of the cornea with fluorescein dye should be carried out on conjunctivitis patients to check for herpes simplex keratitis, particularly in those patients who present with only one infected eye. Herpes simplex virus may also produce follicles in the bulbar and tarsal conjunctiva. Epidemic keratoconjunctivitis is caused by a virus, is spread by aerosol droplets and touching with contaminated hands and clothes, is usually bilateral, and may be severe (**123**).

In severe viral infections, an inflammatory membrane can form on the conjunctiva, particularly on the upper eyelid (**124**).

An antibiotic drop or ointment (tetracycline 1%) may be used every 12 hours for 5 days in both eyes to prevent secondary bacterial infection if the viral infection appears to be severe. The infection usually clears in 10 days. *Do not use corticosteroid drops or ointment to treat a red eye if the diagnosis has not been definitely established.*

Allergic conjunctivitis

Allergic conjunctivitis may be seasonal and may occur in patients with true allergic disease such as bronchial asthma and 'hay fever.' The characteristics of allergic conjunctivitis are as follows:

- A common complaint is itching.
- Visual acuity usually is not affected.
- Enlarged preauricular lymph nodes usually are not present.
- Papillae of vascular reaction are present on the bulbar and tarsal conjunctiva.

Vernal conjunctivitis, a severe form of childhood allergic conjunctivitis, occurs most frequently in prepubertal male children (**125**). Raised conjunctival 'cobblestones' are characteristic. Vernal conjunctivitis at the limbus can cause corneal scarring and, if not stopped, the process can result in central corneal scarring and low vision or blindness.

Topical corticosteroids (drops or ointment) can be used in the management of allergic conjunctivitis in children, but the diagnosis must be certain before therapy is started. *Children who are treated with corticosteroids for vernal conjunctivitis should be examined regularly for complications of steroid use including cataract and ocular hypertension.*

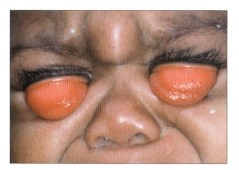

125 Infant with severe allergic conjunctivitis that has everted his eyelids; his eyes were normal.

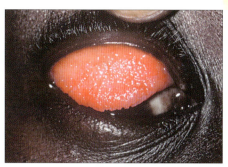

126 Vernal conjunctivitis of upper eyelid.

If possible, identify the substance (animal dander, pollen, or feathers, for example) that is producing the allergy. Identification can be done by skin testing or by selectively removing suspected offending substances from the patient's environment. Removal or control of the offending substance will usually stop the allergic reaction.

Vernal keratoconjunctivitis

Vernal keratoconjunctivitis can be a severe and potentially blinding form of allergic conjunctivitis often beginning at the limbus and progressing on to the peripheral corneae. It is usually bilateral and more common in young boys (**126**). Corticosteroid drops can lessen the symptoms. Corneal ulceration and scarring can result in corneal leucomata in advanced cases. Mast cell stabilizers (sodium chromoglycate, alomide, or nedocromil) are indicated in long-term treatment. For many children, the symptoms and corneal involvement resolve spontaneously in early adulthood. This condition is sometime called 'vernal catarrh' or 'spring catarrh' because it is sometimes seasonal, occurring in springtime.

Mooren's ulcer

This is a peripheral limbal corneal–scleral melting syndrome and not an infection (although frequently it is secondarily infected by bacteria). The corneal stroma is eroded, and the cornea can 'melt' peripherally and extend centrally. Although not common, it should be promptly referred and treated by an ophthalmic surgeon (**127**).

Conjunctival irritation

Dry corneal and conjunctival surfaces will cause a burning or sandy sensation, sometimes reported by the patient as pain. The conjunctiva is irritated and sometimes reddish from mild vascular congestion.

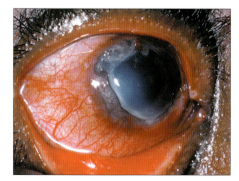

127 Mooren's ulcer (peripheral corneal melting syndrome).

Dry eye may be labeled 'conjunctival irritation' because of the lack of a specific diagnosis. In tropical countries, other causes of conjunctival irritation include excessive exposure to sunlight, wind, dust, and the dry air of desert and high-altitude environments.

Other causes of dry eye

Trachoma can cause alteration or destruction of lubricating glands of the eyelids, resulting in drying of the cornea and conjunctiva. Also, because tear-gland function decreases with age, there is a natural progressive drying of the conjunctiva with aging. In these cases, fluorescein dye will reveal scattered areas of staining on the cornea and conjunctiva.

Dry eye may be treated with isotonic artificial tears, if available. Closure of the lacrimal puncta with thermal cautery can prevent drainage of tears and the increased tear film will moisten the ocular surface, improving symptoms. Temporary punctual plugs may be inserted into the inferior lacrimal puncti to stabilize the tear film.

Epidemic hemorrhagic conjunctivitis

Epidemic hemorrhagic conjunctivitis is a highly infectious viral conjunctivitis with the following symptoms:

- It is usually bilateral.
- Enlarged preauricular lymph nodes usually are not present.
- The cornea usually is not affected.
- Diffuse subconjunctival hemorrhage is present.

Bacterial infection secondary to epidemic hemorrhagic conjunctivitis should be prevented. Tetracycline 1% alone may be applied every 12 hours for 7 days to prevent bacterial infection if discharge is present. *Do not use topical corticosteroid drops.* Corticosteroids are not indicated and complications from them may result.

Purulent (bacterial) conjunctivitis

Bacterial purulent conjunctivitis is characterized by pus (purulent) discharge (**128**). Purulent conjunctivitis can be unilateral or bilateral. Enlarged preauricular lymph nodes usually are not present.

A variety of bacteria may cause purulent conjunctivitis. *Staphylococcus aureus* is responsible for a mild purulent conjunctivitis and blepharitis (infection of the eyelid margins). *Haemophilus* (Koch–Weeks bacillus) and *Moraxella* (Morax–Axenfeld bacillus) are two other types of bacterium that also cause mild purulent conjunctivitis.

Conjunctivitis secondary to coliform (intestinal) bacteria may cause destruction of the cornea if not controlled early in the course of infection. *Pseudomonas* and *Klebsiella* are bacteria that cause severe external ocular infection with corneal destruction.

If the infection is severe (characterized by copious discharge), culture the infection for bacteriological identification and begin treatment in the following sequence:

- With a cotton-tipped applicator, streak the specimen on a blood agar culture plate.
- Streak some of the specimen on a glass slide for a Gram's stain test (see 'Performing a Gram's stain' under 'Bacterial corneal ulcer' below).
- Begin treatment immediately after the culture and streak specimens have been taken using tetracycline 1% ointment three times per day in the affected eye(s).
- Change the antibiotic therapy as needed if results of the culture indicate that the bacteria are not sensitive to tetracycline.

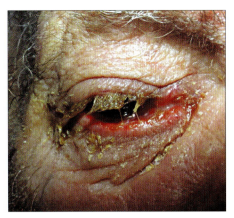

128 Bacterial (purulent) conjunctivitis in an adult.

Gonococcal keratoconjunctivitis in newborns

Ophthalmia neonatorum is a common infection in newborn infants. Several agents may be responsible for ocular infection of the newborn (sexually transmitted *Chlamydia trachomatis*, for example) but the most serious and potentially blinding infection is gonococcal conjunctivitis, which results from contact with *Neisseria gonorrhoeae* in the birth canal. This Gram-negative intracellular *Diplococcus* (GNID) is extremely destructive to ocular tissue, particularly the cornea. Gonococcal conjunctivitis may also occur in children whose eyes have been wiped or cleaned with cloths contaminated with *N. gonorrhoeae*.

The infection is usually bilateral and is characterized by swelling (edema) of the eyelids and heavy discharge of yellow pus. (see Figure 37). The discharge and eyelid swelling appear on the second or third day of life. Prompt treatment is necessary to prevent blindness from corneal scarring or corneal perforation.

Gram's stain for morphology will assist in identification of the bacterium. A specimen should be cultured on blood agar, or even better, chocolate agar medium if possible.

Ceftriaxone antibiotic solution is the drug of choice for gonococcal keratoconjunctivitis. It should be administered one drop hourly around the clock until the infection is cleared. The drug is not widely available in developing countries, but penicillin is usually available.

If ceftriaxone is not available, penicillin drops should be prepared by the pharmacy and then given one drop to each eye hourly around the clock until the infection has cleared. Potential cure of the infection greatly outweighs the risk of conjunctival allergic reaction to topical penicillin. If topical penicillin is not available, tetracycline 1% may be substituted on the same treatment schedule. Injectable (systemic) penicillin should be administered simultaneously to the infant in proper dosage according to weight.

Discharge from the conjunctiva and eyelids should be cleaned with cotton wool and sterile saline every 15 minutes in acute infection. The mother, father, and all their sexual contacts should be examined and treated for active gonorrhea.

Prophylaxis for ophthalmia neonatorum should be available in all nurseries. Silver nitrate 1% (Crede prophylaxis) is difficult to keep in proper solution in hot climates because of evaporation, which makes the solution too concentrated. *Corneal burns and scarring can result from concentrated silver nitrate solution. A solution stronger than 1% and silver nitrate sticks should never be used.* A safer prophylaxis is tetracycline 1% ointment applied to both eyes of all newborn infants at birth. (See also the World Health Organization publication *Conjunctivitis of the Newborn: Prevention and Treatment at the Primary Health Care Level,* listed in Appendix I.)

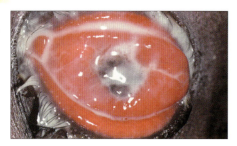

129 Adult with corneal melting and secondary endophthalmitis due to *Neisseria gonorrhoeae*.

Gonococcal keratoconjunctivitis in adults

Gonococcal conjunctivitis and keratoconjunctivitis may occur in adults (**129**). There have been outbreaks of this infection, including periodic epidemics in Africa, that have resulted in permanent blindness and visual disability in many patients. This infection may be spread by poor hygiene and self-inoculation from genital infection. In some areas of rural Africa, urine may be used as an ocular treatment by traditional healers. Urine contaminated with *Neisseria gonorrhoeae* will cause acute gonococcal keratoconjunctivitis (**130**).

Because gonorrhea has become a worldwide public health problem, blindness and low vision from corneal scarring and perforation many increase

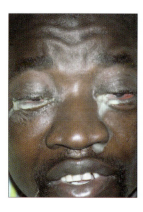

130 Bilateral ocular surface infection secondary to *Neisseria gonorrhoeae* infection.

incidence and prevalence. Early case identification, accurate diagnosis by laboratory investigation and prompt treatment are necessary to prevent corneal destruction from gonococcal keratoconjunctivitis.

Ceftriaxone is the drug of choice (although penicillin is frequently the only drug available). In some regions, the infection may be resistant to penicillin. Where penicillin is effective, properly prepared penicillin drops should be administered to both eyes hourly, and aqueous or procaine penicillin should be administered orally or by injection in appropriate dosage. All sexual contacts should be identified and treated.

Corneal ulcer

A corneal ulcer is an erosion and infection of one or more layers of the cornea. Corneal ulceration nearly always accompanies trachomatous entropion and trichiasis (**131**) and can produce permanent scarring, low vision, and blindness. Bacterial and fungal corneal ulcer are discussed separately here, although the two are often difficult to distinguish clinically except by history, culture of the bacteria causing the infection, and effect of treatment. Early identification and treatment of corneal ulcer will reduce or prevent serious scarring and resultant visual disturbances (**132**).

The cause of corneal ulcer must be determined before proper treatment may be instituted. Common causes include the following:

■ A small corneal epithelial injury (corneal abrasion).
■ Herpes simplex virus infection of the corneal epithelium.
■ Entropion with trichiasis from trachoma (corneal abrasion).
■ Untreated purulent (pus-containing) infections of the ocular surface.

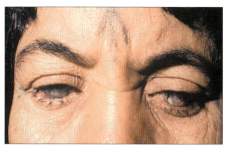

131 Woman bilaterally blind from trachomatous entropion and trichiasis resulting in corneal ulceration and leucomata (WHO).

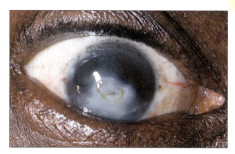

132 Corneal leucoma from ulceration that could have been prevented.

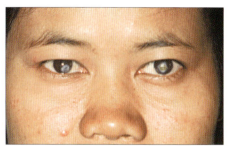

133 Cambodian woman with bilatera leucomata from measles xerophthalmia and cornea ulceration in childhood.

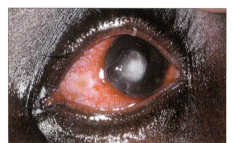

134 Active central corneal ulcer.

A corneal ulcer may be infected with either bacteria or fungi, or both (**133**).

Bacterial corneal ulcer

Common bacterial pathogens in corneal ulcer are as follows:

- *Streptococcus pneumoniae* (*Diplococcus* and *Pneumococcus* are other names in use).
- *Staphylococcus.*
- *Haemophilus.*
- *Moraxella.*

Less common, but very destructive, bacteria that cause corneal ulcers are species of coliform (intestinal) bacteria, including *Pseudomonas* and *Klebsiella.*

Discharge from *Pseudomonas* and *Klebsiella* corneal ulcers is thick, heavy, and greenish in color. If coliform bacterial infection is suspected, treatment should be begun immediately because of the highly destructive nature of these bacteria.

Diagnosis

Bacterial corneal ulcer can occur anywhere on the cornea. It appears as a whitish or yellowish defect, or depression, in the cornea (**134**). A patient with a corneal ulcer will likely complain of pain, tearing, and loss of vision. Additional findings include:

- Purulent discharge is usually present.
- The conjunctiva is infected (reddish from vascular reaction) and irritated.

- Abnormal cells may be visible in the anterior chamber with the slit lamp. If present, these cells layer out in the inferior anterior chamber to form a hypopyon.
- Ciliary flush (blood vessel injection in the sclera at the limbus) may be present. Ciliary flush can be a sign of several types of inflammation: keratitis (inflammation of the cornea, including corneal ulcer); iritis (inflammation of the iris); cyclitis (inflammation of the ciliary body); and iridocyclitis (combined inflammation of the iris and ciliary body). Ciliary flush in corneal ulcer is secondary to keratitis and possibly secondary uveitis (inflammation of any part of the uvea). (See also Appendix A, Diagnosis of the red eye.)

Performing a Gram's stain

Gram's stain will yield valuable information about the morphology and identity of the bacterial infection. The following steps detail how to obtain a Gram's stain:

1. Streak a swab specimen on a clean glass slide, stain with methyl violet for 1 minute, and then wash with water.

2. Flood the slide with iodine for 1 minute and then wash with water.

3. Flood the slide with acetone for 10 seconds only, and then wash with water.

4. Flood the slide with carbolfuchsin, allow it to stand for 1 minute, then wash the slide and allow it to air dry.

5. Examine the stain under the microscope. Assistance from a microbiologist may be necessary to interpret the results.

A specimen of the discharge of the ocular ulcer, taken by cotton-tipped applicator under topical corneal anesthesia, should be plated on blood agar medium for culture and analysis of sensitivity to antibiotics. Then, with a surgical blade, or a corneal spatula designed especially for this purpose, scrape a specimen from the ulcer crater and streak it on a glass slide for Gram's stain. (See 'Performing a Gram's stain', below left.) Debride the ulcer with a corneal spatula or a surgical blade. One must be careful not to damage or perforate the cornea at the ulcer site.

Management

Treatment of bacterial corneal ulcer must be prompt and accurate to prevent blindness from corneal scarring or perforation. Treatment should begin immediately before the laboratory results are reported.

The patient should be hospitalized for treatment if possible. Cefazolin (100 mg in 0.5 cc) should be injected into the subconjunctival space. If the ulcer is severe or progressive and especially if coliform bacteria are suspected, the subconjunctival cefazolin may be repeated daily until the laboratory results are known. If cefazolin is not available, gentamicin 0.5 cc may be substituted, although gentamicin is not particularly effective against *Streptococcus pneumoniae.* Gentamicin is widely available in many countries of the developing world.

Topical tetracycline 1% or sulfacetamide 10% with chloramphenicol drops should be administered hourly until there is obvious improvement (less discharge; ulcer smaller). The antibiotic treatment should be changed if the laboratory reports that the bacteria are not sensitive to the antibiotics being used. Atropine 1% drops or ointment should be applied one drop daily to the affected eye.

The eye should not be patched or occluded. Patching an infected eye may in fact worsen the infection by making the eye warmer, moister, and darker – conditions that encourage the growth of bacteria and fungi.

If the ulcer is deep and perforation of the cornea seems to be possible or imminent, the conjunctiva can be surgically extended over the ulcer to seal the potential perforation. Donor corneal tissue from enucleated eyes may be used to cover large ulcers; donor sclera can be used if donor cornea is not available. The ulcer should be as clean as possible when the conjunctival flap or scleral patch is undertaken.

Fungal corneal ulcer

Fungal corneal ulcer (keratomycosis) is less common than bacterial corneal ulcer. It is often misdiagnosed. Fungal corneal ulcer frequently follows injury to the cornea by plant (vegetable) matter, including leaves; chaff from grain seeds, including rice, millet, and maize; and thorns.

Diagnosis

The possibility of fungal corneal ulcer should be suspected if a plant foreign body has been present on the cornea or if the history indicates that the injury was due to plant matter. Patient complaints include loss of vision and pain. Findings may be similar to bacterial conjunctivitis, with purulent discharge, corneal injection, and hypopyon, although corneal and conjunctival inflammation are usually not severe (bacterial corneal ulcer usually causes greater inflammation). Suspect a fungal corneal ulcer if antibiotics used in treatment of a suspected bacterial corneal ulcer appear to have no effect on the infection.

To verify the diagnosis of fungal corneal ulcer, perform a potassium hydroxide evaluation (see above right).

Evaluating a fungal corneal ulcer with potassium hydroxide (KOH)

1 Apply one drop of topical anesthetic to the cornea.

2 Debride the ulcer with a corneal spatula or a dull surgical blade and, using a cotton-tipped applicator, streak the specimen onto a clean glass slide.

3 Instill one drop of KOH solution over the slide specimen.

4 Examine the slide under the microscope immediately. Spores, filaments, and branching forms of fungi will be visible if fungal infection is present.

5 Attempt to grow the fungal specimen on blood agar or special culture medium in the bacteriology laboratory for specific identification.

Management

Fungal corneal ulcer may be chronic and quite difficult to treat. The treatment is specific: ocular antifungal drugs, which are expensive and difficult to obtain, are necessary. If they are not available, a buffered nystatin solution for topical ocular use may be prepared from powder from nystatin tablets or from nystatin vaginal suppositories dissolved in sterile and pH-balanced solution. A pharmacist should assist in preparing a 1% solution.

Nystatin 1% drops are applied hourly to the involved cornea. Nystatin taken orally has very little or no therapeutic effect on fungal corneal ulcer. In addition, one drop of atropine 1% drops or ointment is applied daily to the affected eye.

If nystatin is not available, one drop of povidone iodine solution may be applied to the affected eye every 12 hours. This solution may be effective against fungal ulcers but it may be toxic. If the eye becomes red or irritated, or the cornea becomes cloudy, discontinue povidone iodine.

Keratitis

Keratitis is inflammation or infection of the cornea. Because it can have many different causes, it is seen in a variety of clinical situations. Often the specific etiology cannot be determined.

Etiology
The most common causes of keratitis are chronic irritation (wood smoke from open fires, for example), lack of normal tear secretion, and foreign bodies. A careful examination of the cornea and everted upper eyelid for foreign bodies and abrasion will often reveal the cause of keratitis (see also Chapter 8, Ocular trauma).

Other less common causes are as follows:
- Stromal herpes simplex infection (see below).
- Syphilis (lues).
- Tuberculosis.
- Leprosy.
- Onchocerciasis.
- Trauma (contusion injury to the eyeball).

If keratitis is due to underlying systemic disease, the underlying disease must be accurately diagnosed. Treatment of keratitis secondary to systemic illness depends on managing the underlying disease.

Diagnosis
Presenting signs and symptoms typically include the following:
- Pain and loss of vision.
- Decreased visual acuity.
- Clouding of the cornea.
- Corneal ulceration (if secondarily infected).
- Ciliary flush.
- Bulbar conjunctival injection.
- Scleritis.

In addition, specific diseases show specific findings and will require particular diagnostic protocols, as follows:

- *Syphilis (lues).* In addition to the general physical examination, a serological test will help establish the presence or absence of syphilis. (Sexually transmitted disease, including syphilis, is increasing worldwide, and keratitis secondary to syphilis will likely increase in prevalence.)
- *Tuberculosis.* Tuberculin skin testing and a chest X-ray should be obtained in addition to a physical examination.
- *Leprosy.* Thorough examination of the skin for evidence of leprosy lesions and examination of hands and feet for loss of fingers and toes is necessary. If keratitis is present, iritis or uveitis is also often present.
- *Onchocerciasis.* In certain areas of Africa and Central and South America where onchocerciasis is endemic, a skin snip for microscopic examination for microfilariae is required for patients who present with keratitis. Characteristic skin nodules of onchocerciasis may be present (see Figure 117). Anterior uveitis, although rare in onchocerciasis, may also be present.
- *Trauma.* An accurate medical history can identify an old injury (contusion or foreign body, for example) as a cause of keratitis and corneal edema.

Management
Do not patch or occlude the affected eye if signs of external infection are present. If keratitis is secondary to a systemic disease (syphilis or tuberculosis, for example), the systemic disease should be treated concurrently with treatment of the keratitis.

Anterior uveitis often occurs with keratitis. Atropine 1% drops or ointment should be applied daily to prevent intraocular complications of iritis and uveitis such as posterior synechiae and iris bombé (see Figures 74, 75).

If keratitis is not due to herpes simplex, topical 1% corticosteroid may be given every 6 hours (or more frequently if necessary) to control and reduce corneal inflammation.

Herpes simplex keratitis

The herpes simplex virus initially infects the corneal epithelium and conjunctival epithelium, causing conjunctivitis. Herpes simplex epithelial keratitis can cause low vision and blindness from corneal scarring if not properly managed. The virus can deeply invade the corneal stroma. Destructive bacteria may secondarily infect this deep corneal defect and corneal perforation and corneal perforation and permanent blindness may result. Deep herpes simplex infection will produce a dense corneal scar when healing finally occurs.

Diagnosis

Herpes simplex keratitis should be suspected in any patient who has loss of vision, corneal clouding, and a painful eye. Corneal sensitivity is reduced in herpes simplex infection. Touching the cornea lightly from the temporal side with a pointed wisp of cotton will cause a blink reflex from a healthy, normal cornea. In herpes simplex keratitis, there will be no blink reflex or a reduced blink reflex at best.

Examination reveals decreased visual acuity and (usually) an injected, reddish conjunctiva. A corneal epithelial defect and corneal clouding (edema) may be seen. The cornea and conjunctiva should be stained with sterile fluorescein dye to identify the corneal epithelial defect.

Fluorescein staining may reveal the typical pattern of herpes simplex corneal epithelial infection, the dendritic (branching) pattern (**135**, **136**). No other virus or infection causes this characteristic dendritic pattern. Herpes simplex may also cause other staining patterns such as punctate (dot) staining or large geographic (area) staining.

Management

Topical corticosteroids are contraindicated in epithelial herpes simplex infection. Corticosteroids can cause deeper corneal invasion by the virus, making the infection worse.

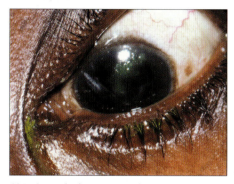

135 Corneal infection secondary to herpes simplex staining with fluorescein dye; note irregular and diffuse edges of staining area.

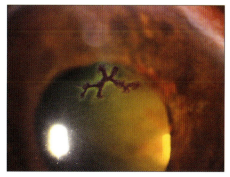

136 Herpes simplex can cause a corneal branching pattern that stains with either Rose Bengal (above) or fluorescein dye. This is diagnostic and is known as dendritic keratitis.

Prompt management of herpes simplex keratitis can prevent low vision and blindness. Idoxuridine (IDU) and trifluridine (Viroptic) are specific medications used in the treatment of herpes simplex keratitis. The patient should receive one drop of idoxuridine or trifluridine every 6 hours for 2 weeks to eliminate remaining virus in the conjunctival and corneal epithelium.

These drugs are expensive and often not available. If both idoxuridine and trifluridine are unavailable, then treat with an antibiotic drop or ointment that does not contain a corticosteroid. Apply one drop every 6 hours to prevent bacterial infection. Atropine 1% should also be given once daily.

Debridement of the affected corneal epithelium with a cotton-tipped applicator, followed by patching until healthy epithelium regenerates is a good alternative to medical treatment of dendritic ulcer.

If deep keratitis (metaherpetic) is secondary to herpes simplex, corticosteroid drops may be used only with the greatest caution and only when used with idoxuridine or trifluridine. *Corticosteroids should never be used if a dendrite in the corneal epithelium is present.*

Other external diseases

Pterygium
Pterygium is a conjunctival growth that extends onto the cornea (**137**). It is common in hot, dry climates. Excessive exposure to sunlight and dry climatic conditions may be factors in pterygium formation.

It occurs most frequently on the nasal conjunctiva and extends onto the cornea. The patient with pterygium should be examined at regular intervals. If the pterygium begins to encroach upon the visual axis and visual acuity is affected, surgical removal should be undertaken. Surgery should include removal of the base of the pterygium, wide resection of surrounding conjunctiva, and thermal cautery of underlying sclera. Because of the high rate of recurrence, a pterygium should not be surgically excised if it extends only 1–2 mm onto the cornea.

Pinguecula
Pinguecula (plural, pingueculae) is a small, raised mound of conjunctiva at the limbus, usually in the nasal limbal position. It can be a precursor of pterygium. Surgical removal is not necessary.

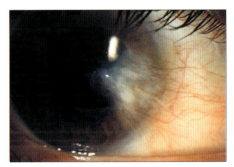

137 Pterygium encroaching on center of cornea and visual axis; pterygium surgery is usually not performed unless growth can be demonstrated or if vision is compromised.

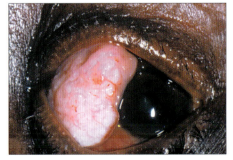

138 Advanced squamous cell carcinoma of the conjunctiva.

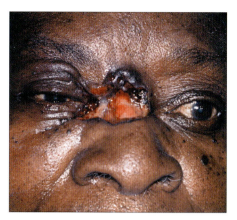

139 Basal cell carcinoma.

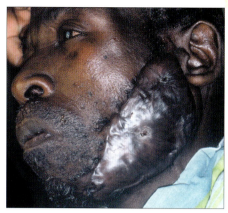

140 Keloid (scar); be cautious about performing eyelid surgery on patients with a history of keloid formation.

Squamous cell carcinoma and basal cell carcinoma

Squamous cell carcinoma (surface cancer) of the conjunctiva is rare. It is thought to be more common in high-altitude climates where sunlight exposure is great. Rapid growth of squamous cell carcinoma in a young person suggests underlying HIV/AIDS infection.

Squamous cell carcinoma may resemble pterygium or pinguecula but may occur anywhere on the conjunctiva (**138**). Large blood vessels may occur around this conjunctival tumor. It often appears inflamed and irritated.

Surgical removal of this tumor and microscopic identification should be carried out as a surgical emergency. Squamous cell carcinoma of the conjunctiva can invade the orbit and eyeball and is life threatening if not managed properly .

Basal cell carcinoma can occur on facial skin and can be aggressively invasive. It should be surgically biopsied and excised (**139**).

Keloid

Keloid results from excessive skin and subcutaneous healing reaction from trauma or surgery (**140**). Any patient who needs ocular adnexal or eyelid surgery and who presents with keloid formation should be referred to an ophthalmologist for evaluation and treatment.

Conjunctival pigmentation

Excessive pigmentation, darkening of the conjunctiva, and pigmented conjunctival spots are common. No treatment is necessary for diffuse (scattered) pigmentation. A densely pigmented spot may be a conjunctival nevus.

A raised, deeply pigmented, and enlarging spot may be a conjunctival melanoma, a rare but highly malignant tumor. It should be surgically excised immediately with generous surgical margins and microscopically identified.

Phlyctenule

A phlyctenule is a raised, inflamed spot at the junction of the sclera and cornea. Phlyctenules may be secondary to an immune reaction. They may be caused by tuberculosis, and clinical investigation should include tuberculin skin testing.

A phlyctenule may also be caused by *Staphylococcus*. If discharge is present, do culture and sensitivity testing and treat accordingly.

Scleritis

Scleritis is a pinkish/reddish patch that appears to lie deep to the conjunctiva at any position on the sclera and that is usually tender to the touch. The patient may complain of pain and irritation, but visual acuity is rarely affected. If the area where redness of the sclera is present is touched by the examiner with the patient's eyelids closed and tenderness is found, scleritis is probably present.

Blood vessel congestion in the conjunctiva may be distinguished from scleritis by a simple test, as follows: Place one drop of topical anesthetic on the eye. Move the conjunctiva just overlying the redness with a cotton-tipped applicator. If the red patch moves with the applicator, it is in the conjunctiva; if the red patch does not move, it is in the sclera.

Scleritis may be a sign of systemic disease, particularly rheumatoid arthritis. Specific laboratory tests are required to establish this diagnosis.

Scleritis can be treated with topical corticosteroids. The patient must be followed carefully, however, because chronic scleritis can result in scleral thinning and perforation.

Blepharitis

Inflammation or infection of the eyelids or eyelid margins (blepharitis) rarely causes visual disturbance. Erythromycin or tetracycline 1% ointment applied to the eyelid margins and cleaning the eyelid margins with a cotton-tipped applicator and mild non-detergent soap and clean water every 12 hours for 1 week will usually clear the infection. *Staphylococcus* is a common cause of blepharitis.

Phthirus pubis, the crab louse, may attach to eyelashes and lay eggs, causing blepharitis. Magnification with the slit lamp is required to make this identification. A scalp louse disinfectant applied carefully with a cotton-tipped applicator to

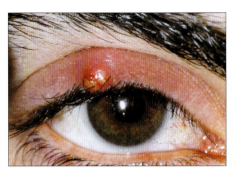

141 External hordeolum (stye).

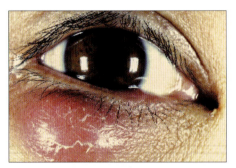

142 Chalazion.

the eyelid margins only, or physostigmine ointment applied every 12 hours to the eyelid margins for 2 days, will cure the infestation. Removal of the crab lice and eggs with fine forceps under slit-lamp magnification is an effective control.

Hordeolum

Hordeolum, or stye, is a small abscess in the eyelid margin, usually secondary to *Staphylococcus* (**141**). Warm compresses and tetracycline 1% ointment every 12 hours for 1 week usually cure this infection.

Chalazion

Chalazion results from a blocked duct in an eyelid gland. It presents as a pea-sized lump on the eyelid surface. Some chalazia may be inflamed or infected (**142, 143**).

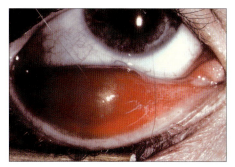

143 Inflamed chalazion.

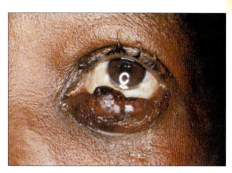

144 Kaposi's sarcoma of the lower eyelid secondary to HIV/AIDS.

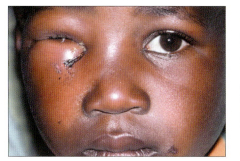

145 Preseptal cellulitis – an ophthalmic emergency.

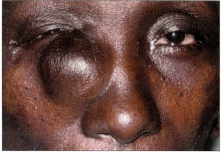

146 Advanced dacryocystitis from obstructed naso-lacrimal duct.

Surgical removal (incision and curettage) under local anesthesia from the tarsal (inner) aspect of the eyelid can be carried out. Chalazion should not be confused with Kaposi's sarcoma of the eyelids (**144**), sometimes a presentation of HIV/AIDS.

Eyelid infection

Penetration, abrasion, or contusion to the eyelids can lead to pyogenic (pus-producing) infection. Infection in the inner tissue of the eyelids may result in cellulitis, a potentially severe infection. Eyelid cellulitis (**145**) should be suspected where there is marked swelling of the eyelids. The eyelids may be warm to the touch, reddish, and swollen. This infection is an ophthalmic emergency and should be treated intensively with appropriate antibiotics by a specialist.

Lacrimal disease

Infection or obstruction of the lacrimal system can obstruct normal tear drainage, causing excessive tearing. Tearing is common in infants if the nasolacrimal duct is not patent (open) at birth. Most blocked nasolacrimal ducts will open spontaneously before 1 year of age. Probing may be necessary to open the nasolacrimal duct after 1 year of age.

External infection, including trachoma, may produce canaliculitis (infection of the canaliculi) and dacryocystitis (infection of the lacrimal sac) (**146**). In adults, control of infection and then probing of the lacrimal drainage system will identify the site of blockage. The obstruction may be opened with further probing of the drainage system. Surgery may be required to re-establish tear drainage. Lacrimal drainage

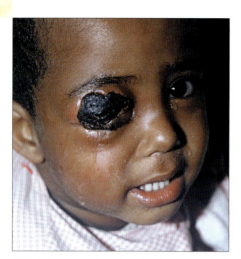

147 Cutaneous anthrax (wool-sorter's disease) of the upper eyelid in an Ethiopian child.

surgery is not a high priority when many surgically curable blind patients are awaiting sight-restoring operations.

Anthrax

Pulmonary and cutaneous anthrax (also known as wool-sorter's disease) is caused by the bacterium *Bacillus anthracis*. Although rare, it can occur among pastoral peoples who keep and herd livestock, particularly sheep. Pulmonary anthrax can be fatal. Cutaneous antrax (**147**) can affect the skin of the face and eyelids. Patients with suspected anthrax should be referred for medical and possibly surgical treatment, particularly if scarring or retraction of the eyelids has occurred or if the infection appears to be systemic.

12

Other blinding disorders

If your eye is sound, your whole body will be full of light.
Matthew 6:22

Although just two ocular diseases – cataract and glaucoma – are responsible for about 60% of world blindness, a variety of other disorders account for the remaining 40% (**148**). Worldwide, age-related macular degeneration (AMD) ranks third (9%), though it is the leading cause of blindness in industrialized countries. Trachoma, discussed in Chapter 7, accounts for nearly 4% of blindness and low vision. Several other common blinding disorders are presented in this chapter. The text does not attempt to include all possible remaining causes; the publications listed in Appendix J will provide more comprehensive information about these and other causes of blindness.

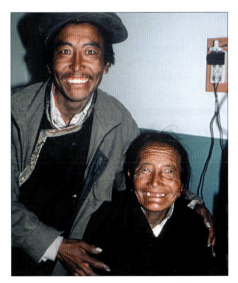

148 Avoidable blindness is a public health problem in Tibet, with cataract the major cause of blindness there.

Diseases of the ocular fundus

The diagnosis of diseases of the posterior segment and ocular fundus depends on careful examination with the ophthalmo-scope. Direct ophthalmoscopy can be learned with practice; indirect ophthal-moscopy, needed for examining the retinal periphery and for eyes with opacities of the media, requires either a slit lamp or special lenses and a headlamp, and demands considerable training and much practice to master.

Ophthalmoscopy should be performed on all patients with unexplained visual loss. Open-angle glaucoma (see Chapter 6) is the most common disease with fundus findings responsible for blindness in most developing nations.

In comparison, diabetes mellitus, with its associated damage to the retina (retinopathy) and vitreous, is a major cause of blindness in industrialized countries. Diabetes mellitus and diabetic retinopathy are also increasing in prevalence in the developing world. The optic nerve head (optic disc) should always be examined during ophthalmoscopy, because glaucoma may be present even in the presence of other fundus disease.

Diabetic retinopathy

Diabetic retinopathy is responsible for almost 5% of visual impairment across the globe and, as older age groups among populations become larger, is growing in prevalence. Diabetic retinopathy can produce growth of blood vessels in the retina and vitreous, causing hemorrhage and retinal detachment. Medical control of diabetes mellitus with oral medications or insulin is essential. The growth of abnormal retinal vessels can be controlled by treatment (photocoagulation) with the argon laser instrument. The argon laser can also be used to control leakage of serous fluid in the central retina (which causes retinal thickening) by applying multiple laser burns in a grid pattern, called a focal grid.

Every diabetes mellitus patient should have regular funduscopy performed by a skilled eye health care worker, preferably once a year. The pupils should be dilated for the examination and the central, mid, and far retinal peripheries should be examined for signs of diabetic retinopathy.

Retinopathy from diabetes has no symptoms until leakage from blood vessels begins to occur. Serous fluid leakage in the macular area may cause decreased central vision. Bleeding from new blood vessel formation (neovascularization) and from tiny swellings of the retinal veins (microaneurysms) may be the first signs of retinopathy from diabetes. Intraretinal

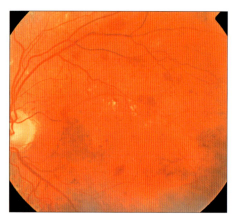

149 Background retinopathy in diabetes mellitus. Note blood vessel abnormalities with swollen small veins and bleeding in the retina (intraretinal hemorrhage).

hemorrhages may occur. Changes in the retina only are referred to as background diabetic retinopathy (BDR) (**149**). There is no pain unless glaucoma with high pressure occurs simultaneously.

When bleeding occurs into the vitreous from background retinopathic changes, neovascularization may proceed, eventually resulting in retinal detachment and irreversible blindness. The progression of blood vessel growth in the retina and growth in the vitreous is known as proliferative diabetic retinopathy (PDR). Proliferative diabetic retinopathy is a dangerous sign, and if detected, should be managed immediately by a vitro-retinal specialist.

As more diabetes mellitus patients survive because of better treatment, blindness and low vision from ocular complications will become more prevalent worldwide.

Macular degeneration

Degeneration of the macula, the central area of the retina, usually occurs in older patients, but certain types of hereditary macular degeneration may occur in young patients. Age-related macular degeneration (AMD) is much more common than hereditary macular degeneration. AMD is a leading cause of blindness in the industrialized world, and is increasing in prevalence in the developing world.

Macular degeneration affects central visual acuity, whereas peripheral vision is preserved; therefore, visual acuity measurement is a good indicator of possible macular degeneration. An excellent clinical test for macular degeneration is the Amsler Grid. This consists of a central fixation point and straight lines arranged in vertical and horizontal configuration to form squares (see page 272). The patient is tested one eye at a time (right, then left). The grid is held at a distance of approximately 20 cm (reading distance) under normal lighting conditions. The patient is asked to look at the central fixation point and describe what is seen around it. If curved or irregular lines are seen, or there are blank areas, then macular degeneration might be present.

Macular degeneration should be suspected in adults with reduced visual acuity and clear ocular media. (Open-angle glaucoma is another common cause of blindness and low vision in adults that should be suspected when the ocular media are clear and peripheral or central vision is reduced.)

Macular degeneration is usually bilateral. A simple classification of macular degeneration is (1) dry (atrophic) macular degeneration, and (2) wet (serous) macular degeneration. The macula loses its normal bright reflex and becomes either darkly pigmented (hyperpigmented) or lightly pigmented (hypopigmented). This is usually the dry or atrophic type (**150**).

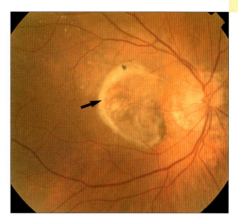

150 Macular degeneration displaying findings of both atrophic ("dry" type) and disciform scar (arrow) from old vascular involvement ("wet" type). Note loss of normal macular structure, absent foveal reflex, and light areas (depigmentation) in macula. No serous fluid is present.

The area of macular degeneration may be elevated if abnormal blood vessels grow into the macular area and leak fluid (wet or serous type). Special low vision aids, including spectacles, can improve vision, particularly for reading and near work. (See Chapter 14.) Poor nutrition may play a role in age-related macular degeneration. Some studies have shown that supplementing the diets of patients with atrophic macular degeneration with certain micronutrient antioxidants (vitamins A, C, E and zinc, for example) might slow the progression of their macular degeneration.

Reduction or loss of macular vision in infancy may result in nystagmus (involuntary, rapid, rhythmic movement of the eyeball). Nystagmus may also be caused by numerous neurological disorders in children and adults.

Retinal detachment

Retinal detachment (or retinal separation), although not one of the major causes of blindness worldwide, is nevertheless a significant cause of monocular blindness.

It can occur without any apparent cause or reason. Retinal detachment frequently occurs following ocular trauma and also is associated with diabetes mellitus. It can occur after cataract surgery.

Symptoms of retinal detachment are 'lightning flashes' of light or 'sparks' in the visual field, clouding of vision, or a 'curtain' across part of the visual field. Pain is not a finding in retinal detachment.

When retinal detachment is suspected, the patient should be examined by someone skilled in indirect ophthalmoscopy. Viewed by ophthalmoscopy, the retina appears whitish and uneven in the area where it is separated from its attachments in the ocular fundus. Surgical repair should be performed as soon as possible. Acute retinal detachment is a surgical emergency.

Retinal degeneration

Retinal degenerations are diseases for which there is no effective treatment. They usually result in progressive and permanent loss of vision. Several types are hereditary. Retinal degenerations often affect the peripheral retina before the central retina and macula are affected. Indirect ophthalmoscopy is usually necessary to establish the diagnosis.

The retina in malaria

Malaria is a major cause of death in children in tropical countries, particularly in Africa. In children who are unconscious (in coma) from febrile illness, malaria – particularly falciparum malaria – should be suspected in areas where the disease is known to occur. In cerebral malaria, flat, white retinal patches, together with whitish or orange blood vessels, often appear in the macular area and the retinal periphery. The pupils should be fully dilated with mydriatic drops to observe these signs with an ophthalmoscope. The presence of these signs is usually indicative of cerebral malaria, a commonly fatal disease in children.

Optic atrophy

Open-angle glaucoma, one of the world's major causes of blindness, is the most common etiology of optic atrophy. Other causes include the following:

■ Injuries, such as severe blunt injury to the orbit and eyeball.
■ Onchocerciasis.
■ Intracranial mass. (If an intracranial mass causes increased intracranial pressure, papilledema – swelling of the optic nerve – may occur initially, followed by optic atrophy.)
■ Vascular disease that reduces blood supply to the optic nerve.

Toxic optic atrophy can follow the ingestion of impure distilled spirits. It should be suspected where distilled spirits are produced locally. Methyl alcohol (wood alcohol) is toxic to the nervous system, including the brain and optic nerve. Unexplained bilateral optic atrophy may be due to poisoning (toxic cause), and methyl alcohol poisoning from impure homemade drinking spirits should be suspected as a cause if other causes do not seem to be possibilities.

Strabismus (squint)

Strabismus, or squint, refers to the condition of the eyes being misaligned so that only one eye at a time fixes on the visual target. Strabismus should be suspected when the light reflexes from a flashlight (torch) are not centered on the corneas (in the centers of the pupils) (**151**). If left untreated, strabismus can produce monocular low vision or blindness.

When the eyes are looking straight ahead, they are in primary position. *Exotropia* ('wall eyes') refers to outward deviation of an eye when the eyes are in primary position; *esotropia* ('crossed eyes') is inward deviation. *Hypertropia* refers to

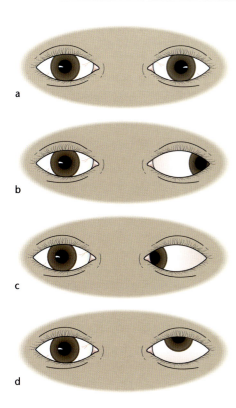

151 Strabismus and corneal light reflex:
primary position (a); exotropia (b); esotropia (c);
hypertropia (d).

loss of two lines of vision on the visual
acuity chart while wearing best-corrected
spectacles as compared with the other eye,
in the absence of ocular disease or injury.
Only rarely does strabismus result in loss
of vision or amblyopia in both eyes. It is a
common cause of monocular low vision.

The ability of the eye to see properly
develops early in life. Maximum binocular
eyesight is possible only if both eyes are
aligned correctly and track together. When
an eye is misaligned, it fails to 'learn to see'
(amblyopia) and maximum vision does not
develop. If amblyopia has not been
corrected by age 6 years it is unlikely that
any treatment after that age will restore
vision to the amblyopic eye; therefore, an
infant or child with strabismus should be
treated as soon as the diagnosis is made.
The fixing eye (the eye with better visual
acuity) should be occluded, or patched,
6 days per week while the child is awake.
It should be left unpatched the seventh day.
Patching the better eye forces the deviating
eye to develop better visual acuity.

A refraction is necessary. In infants and
children, the most accurate method is with
retinoscopy. The retinoscope is an instrument for determining the refractive state of
an eye using various lenses against the
retinal red reflex. The examination is done
under cycloplegia (pupil dilated and fixed
and the ciliary body at rest to eliminate
accommodation) with atropine 1%.

If the child is old enough to cooperate
with visual testing, visual acuity is measured with a testing chart designed for use
with illiterate patients, such as a Landolt
ring C chart (see Figure 11) or E chart (see
inside back cover). With infants, vision may
be assessed by testing the ability of the
child to maintain fixation on a near target,
preferably a flashlight (torch). If the
squinting eye can hold fixation, then visual
acuity is assumed to be normal, near
normal, or has potential to be normal.

upward deviation of one eye. Hypertropia
is more difficult to diagnose than exotropia
or esotropia because the degree of
deviation may be small and the eyes may
appear to be aligned normally.

Primary strabismus

Strabismus is usually primary; that is, it
occurs early in childhood without any
apparent cause. It may be inherited and
several children in the same family can
develop strabismus early in childhood
within the first months or years of life.
In children, the eye that is constantly misaligned fails to develop the ability to see
clearly and becomes amblyopic.
Amblyopia, or 'lazy eye,' is defined as the

When visual acuity in both eyes is equal, or nearly so, corrective extraocular muscle surgery should be performed to realign the eyes. The earlier the surgery is undertaken, the better the chance of preventing amblyopia and preserving useful vision. Infants only a few months of age can undergo extraocular muscle surgery under general anesthesia. Strabismus surgery should be performed as soon as possible on patients for whom follow-up care is difficult. An occlusion (patching) program can be successful only if the patient is examined frequently and only if the parents understand the reasons for treatment.

Secondary strabismus

Secondary strabismus may follow direct trauma to one or both eyes. Injuries that cause opacities of the media in childhood, especially injuries that produce corneal scars or cataracts, are likely to cause secondary strabismus. Particularly in adults, secondary strabismus may also be due to a cranial nerve palsy from any of the following conditions:

- Head injury.
- Intracranial mass (brain tumor or abscess, for example).
- Vascular accident (stroke).
- Diabetes mellitus.
- Vascular disease.
- Heart disease.
- Systemic hypertension.

If secondary strabismus is suspected, the patient should be evaluated by an internal medicine specialist and neurologist.

Strabismus in a child may be caused by an opacity of the media or even by an intraocular tumor. *Be aware of retinoblastoma, a highly malignant tumor occurring in children under 5 years of age*. Retinoblastoma may present with a white pupil (leukocoria) (see Figure 35).

Uveitis associated with systemic diseases

Many systemic diseases may be associated with uveitis, which results in visual disability and blindness. Determining an etiology for uveitis is not always possible. Uveitis may occur with onchocerciasis (Chapter 9), tuberculosis, leprosy (Chapter 10), syphilis (lues), AIDS, and other systemic diseases, which are global public health problems.

Anterior uveitis is defined as inflammation and reaction of the iris and/or ciliary body. Typical symptoms of anterior uveitis include pain, photophobia, decreased vision, and tearing. Signs of anterior uveitis, no matter what the cause, include scleral blood vessel congestion at the limbus (ciliary flush), corneal haziness due to edema, conjunctival injection, abnormal (irregular) pupillary shape and size indicating posterior synechiae (**152**; see also Figure 74), and sluggish pupillary reaction to light. Peripheral anterior synechiae (PAS) and iris bombé may result (if 360° posterior synechiae are present).

Cells and flare may be seen in the anterior chamber upon slit-lamp examination. Deep (interstitial) keratitis may be present. Keratic (corneal) precipitates, or KPs, may be found on the corneal endothelium. The KPs appear as spots, or dots, adhering to the inner surface of the cornea. Magnification with a slit lamp is required to visualize them, but heavy deposits on the corneal endothelium may be seen with the aid of a hand-held magnifying lens.

Posterior uveitis involves the choroid and the retina overlying it (chorioretinitis). Posterior uveitis is usually painless and the only symptom may be loss of visual field and decreased central acuity due to cells and protein in the vitreous. Ophthalmoscopy, particularly indirect ophthalmoscopy, is necessary to diagnose posterior uveitis.

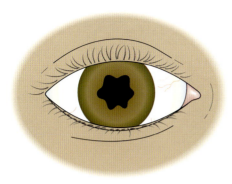

152 Irregular pupil indicating posterior synechiae.

Tuberculosis

Uveitis should be suspected in all tuberculosis patients who complain of eye problems. To diagnose tuberculosis, sputum containing the mycobacterial organism is stained with the acid-fast technique and identified. Tuberculosis skin testing should also be carried out. X-ray examination of the chest can confirm the diagnosis of tuberculosis if a lung lesion is present.

Low vision and blindness from tuberculous uveitis can be delayed or prevented. Accurate diagnosis of tuberculosis and control of the disease by proper medical therapy are of the utmost importance in controlling uveitis secondary to tuberculosis.

If the tuberculosis organism infects the lymph nodes of the neck, a necklace of skin depigmentation and nodular lumps may appear. This sign is known as scrofula.

Systemic treatment of tuberculosis should accompany treatment of tuberculous keratitis and uveitis. Treating the primary disease lessens the severity and intraocular damage from tuberculous uveitis. Tuberculous chorioretinitis and subsequent scarring can result in severe visual loss or blindness. In addition to treating the systemic disease, topical atropine 1% drops or ointment and corticosteroids in appropriate dosages are necessary to control uveitis.

Leprosy

All leprosy patients with ocular complaints should be carefully examined for evidence of uveitis. (See also more detailed discussion of leprosy in Chapter 10.) Multibacillary leprosy is more frequently responsible for low vision and blindness from uveitis than paucibacillary leprosy. The signs and symptoms of leprosy uveitis are similar to those of tuberculosis uveitis. The management is the same.

Syphilis

Keratitis and uveitis may be associated with syphilis (lues). Ocular findings in syphilitic uveitis are similar to those of tuberculous uveitis. Syphilitic uveitis may result in visual disability and blindness. All patients with confirmed syphilis and ocular complaints should be examined for evidence of keratitis and uveitis.

A serology test for syphilis (a VDRL or Kahn test) should be performed in all patients with severe uveitis or keratitis. Once the diagnosis of syphilis has been made, systemic treatment with the appropriate dosage of penicillin should be started. Ocular complications of syphilis are treated at the same time. The treatment of corneal inflammation and uveitis from syphilis is the same as for keratitis and uveitis secondary to other etiologies – topical atropine 1% and topical corticosteroids. All persons with whom the patient has had sexual contact should be examined and tested for syphilis: those testing positive should undergo treatment.

Acquired immunodeficiency syndrome (AIDS)

Acquired immunodeficiency syndrome (AIDS) has become a serious public health problem. The human immunodeficiency virus (HIV), which causes AIDS, is transmitted by sexual contact, blood products, and contaminated needles of drug abusers, and by improper, non-sterile procedures of hospitals and clinics. AIDS may affect multiple organ systems, including the visual system, by opportunistic diseases that attack the body because of its weakened immune system.

Patients with AIDS may present with visual disturbances secondary to uveitis. Posterior uveitis, severe anterior uveitis, or panuveitis (inflammation of iris, ciliary body, and choroid) may occur with AIDS in one or both eyes simultaneously.

Herpes zoster of the first division of the trigeminal (fifth cranial) nerve, also known as 'shingles,' can accompany AIDS-related decreased visual acuity and uveitis, particularly in young patients. AIDS should be suspected in any patient who presents with herpes zoster and/or uveitis (**153**) or shingles.

Other clinical signs that may be associated with AIDS include the following:

- Weight loss.
- Muscle wasting.
- Diarrhea.
- Respiratory infection.
- Neurological signs.

Disseminated and severe chorioretinitis may occur in HIV/AIDS infection, rapidly compromising vision and causing blindness.

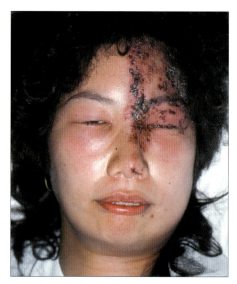

153 Herpes zoster ophthalmicus. HIV/AIDS should always be considered in the differential diagnosis of HZO infection.

Evaluation and management of uveitis

Evaluation

Consider in the diagnosis the following:

- Onchocerciasis (where endemic).
- Tuberculosis.
- Leprosy.
- Syphilis.
- HIV/AIDS.
- Lens-induced causes (leaking hypermature cataract).
- Ocular contusion injury (a careful history from the patient is necessary to determine if trauma is a possible etiology).
- Rheumatoid arthritis.
- Sympathetic ophthalmia in an otherwise normal eye following penetrating injury to the other eye (although rare, sympathetic ophthalmia is often blinding when it does occur).

Relevant investigations to pursue include:
- Three consecutive sputa for acid-fast stain (tuberculosis).
- Examination of the skin for the nodules and depigmentation of onchocerciasis or for evidence of multibacillary or paucibacillary leprosy.
- Skin-snip examination for microfilariae (onchocerciasis).
- Serological testing (syphilis/AIDS).
- Examination of the anterior chamber and lens with the slit lamp (hyper-mature cataract).

Management

It is often not possible to determine the etiology of uveitis. If the etiology is known, uveitis may be managed as follows:

- Atropine 1% drops or ointment every 12 hours to affected eyes for 3 days for full pupillary dilation to prevent posterior synechiae.
- Topical 0.5 or 1% corticosteroid drops or ointment every 6 hours; subconjunctival corticosteroids for eyes that are severely inflamed and that require a high corticosteroid level to reduce inflammation. Be cautious in using topical or subconjunctival cortico-steroids; check for contraindications (herpes simplex or fungal keratitis).
- Intraocular pressure monitoring. Ocular hypertension and secondary glaucoma are frequent complications of uveitis. Intraocular pressure should be monitored daily for inpatients and as often as necessary for outpatients on uveitis treatment.

Proper diagnosis (particularly of systemic disease, if present) and appropriate management can prevent ocular damage and visual loss from uveitis, which can result in secondary cataracts, glaucoma, or scarring of the cornea and retina.

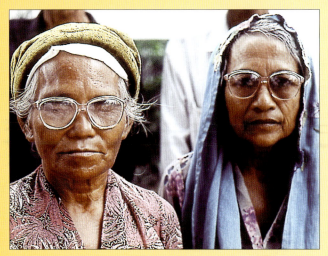
Women receiving new spectacles at a clinic in rural Bangladesh.

13

Refractive errors

Millions of people are blind because they don't have access to spectacles.
Vision 2020, WHO and IAPB

*Simple refractive errors are associated potentially with good vision
and require no treatment apart from their optical correction.*
Sir Stewart Duke-Elder

The precise number of people blind from uncorrected refractive errors is not known. WHO estimates that severe refractive error accounts for 5 million blind. In addition, there are approximately 124 million people with low vision due to refractive error. Recent studies have confirmed the global burden of uncorrected refractive error. Correcting refractive error is cost-effective and significantly improves quality of life. The majority of people with refractive error in the developing world are uncorrected with spectacles or any optical device.

This chapter provides basic definitions of terms used in refraction and optics, descriptions of useful refraction tools, and practical tips for performing refraction. The following material is not meant as a substitute for a manual on refraction. Instead, it is an introduction to simple refraction techniques, terminology, and resources. Expert refraction is learned through careful instruction from a thoughtful teacher and by continuous practice.

Refractive error

A refractive error is an optical defect of the eye that prevents light from being brought to a sharp focus by the cornea and lens onto the retina (**154**). Varying degrees of decreased vision, low vision, or blindness result from refractive error, depending on the type and severity. If a refractive error is present, it is usually present in both eyes, often to nearly the same degree. Certain refractive errors can be hereditary.

Emmetropia is a term that describes an eye with no refractive error. *Ametropia* describes an eye with any form of refractive error. Types of ametropia include myopia, hyperopia, presbyopia, astigmatism, aphakia, and pseudophakia.

Myopia

Myopic people are said to be 'shortsighted' or 'nearsighted' because they have good vision at close range but poor distance vision. In myopia, the image is brought to a focus in front of the retina. The problem is that the eyeball is too long for the refractive power of the lens and the cornea. If myopia develops in childhood, it usually

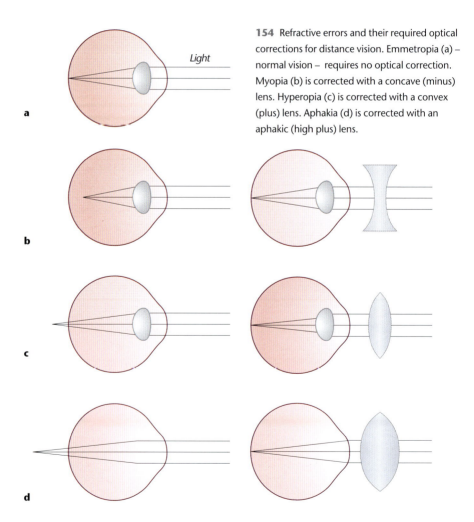

154 Refractive errors and their required optical corrections for distance vision. Emmetropia (a) – normal vision – requires no optical correction. Myopia (b) is corrected with a concave (minus) lens. Hyperopia (c) is corrected with a convex (plus) lens. Aphakia (d) is corrected with an aphakic (high plus) lens.

Light

a

b

c

d

progresses until body growth is completed. When adult growth stops, the eyeball usually ceases to grow lengthwise, and worsening of myopia then slows or stops.

Myopia may also develop in adulthood with early cataract, when the lens thickens and causes light to be focused in front of the retina. High myopia, or myopia greater than 6 diopters, can be progressive throughout life. Retinal detachment or retinal separation is more frequent in people with high myopia. Myopia is corrected with concave, or minus, lenses.

Hyperopia

Hyperopic people are said to be 'farsighted' because they have good vision at distance but poor vision at close range. In hyperopia, the eyeball is too short for the power of the lens and cornea. Most children are hyperopic (so-called *physiological hyperopia*, because hyperopia is normal in childhood), and the degree of hyperopia gradually lessens as the child approaches adolescence. With aging and gradual loss of accommodation, hyperopia causes symptoms of eye strain (discomfort) and decreased visual acuity. Primary angle-closure glaucoma is more frequent in people with hyperopia. Hyperopia is corrected with convex, or plus, lenses.

Presbyopia

Presbyopia occurs as a result of the normal aging process. The lens loses its elasticity with age, and in time can no longer change shape (accommodate) well enough to focus the image on the retina at close range. Most people first notice this problem when presbyopia creates difficulty with reading. In an emmetropic person, this begins to occur at approximately age 40 years and is progressive thereafter. Decreased visual acuity and ocular discomfort when reading are symptoms. Presbyopia occurs earlier than age 40 years in hyperopic eyes and later than age

40 years in myopic eyes. Presbyopia is corrected with convex lenses to improve near vision. A presbyopic person who wears spectacles to improve distance vision will require a second pair of spectacles for near vision, or bifocal lenses can be provided.

Astigmatism

The normal central corneal surface is spherical, similar to the surface of a ball. If it is non-spherical, or astigmatic, like the surface of an egg, the image is brought to focus at two different points. Astigmatism is corrected by compound non-spherical (cylindrical) lenses.

Aphakia

A normal eye with the lens in place is phakic; if the lens has been removed (cataract extraction), the eye is aphakic. The optical power must be replaced after intracapsular cataract extraction (ICCE) with either a spectacle lens or contact lens. This requires a high plus (convex) lens. Cataract spectacles (aphakic spectacles) are still used in some regions where extracapsular cataract extraction (ECCE) with intraocular lens (IOL) implantation is not routinely performed. The contact lens and the intraocular lens (IOL) implant are also used to correct vision in the aphakic eye. Vision in an uncorrected aphakic eye is usually classified as 'blindness' as defined by the World Health Organization (Appendix F), because without optical correction, aphakic vision is poor.

Pseudophakia

Pseudophakia is the condition of an eye that has had an IOL implanted after a cataract has been removed. The IOL does not accommodate (focus) like a normal crystalline lens, so spectacles are usually required to correct visual acuity to best possible levels at both distance and near.

Optics

The diopter is the basic unit of lens power. A lens that has 1 diopter of power will bring light from a distant object into focus at a distance of 1 m from the lens. The stronger the lens, the shorter its focal length. A 2-diopter lens focuses light at a distance of 0.5 m (50 cm). To calculate the focal length of a lens, divide the power of the lens into 1.00 m (100 cm). For example, the focal length of a 5-diopter lens is 20 cm (100 cm divided by 5 diopters = 20 cm).

Refractive errors are described in diopters as follows:

- The refractive error of myopic eyes is given in minus (–) diopters because concave, or minus, lenses are required for correction of myopia.
- The refractive error of hyperopic eyes is expressed in plus (+) diopters because convex, or plus, lenses are required to correct hyperopia.
- The amount of presbyopia is expressed in plus diopters because convex lenses are required to correct visual acuity at close range. Presbyopic correction supplements the accommodative power of the eyes.

Equipment and instruments

The following tools are useful for determining refractive error:

- *Visual acuity chart* (see Figure 11) and near visual acuity card (see inside front cover of this book).
- *Pinhole*. The pinhole test should be performed on all patients with decreased visual acuity (see Chapter 16). In this test, the patient with decreased vision is asked to look through a pinhole device; if the patient can read at least one line better on the visual acuity chart, it is likely that decreased visual acuity is due to a refractive error. Visual acuity in a patient with superficial corneal scarring or posterior subcapsular cataract may also improve with the pinhole test. (See Chapter 3 for instructions for manufacturing a simple pinhole testing device.)
- *Lensometer.* The lensometer determines the power of an optical lens. The power of the spectacles a patient is wearing can be determined, and this current refraction can be used as a starting point for a new refraction. The lensometer is a valuable instrument for the refraction clinic.
- *Trial lens set.* Such a set contains loose minus and plus lenses, cylindrical lenses, and trial frames for children and adults. It may also contain a pinhole testing device.
- *Phoropter.* A self-contained instrument for refraction, the phoropter contains necessary lenses on dials for use in refraction.
- *Retinoscope.* Using the retinoscope light, a skilled refractionist can determine the refractive error objectively by streak retinoscopy (see below).
- *Autorefractor.* Automatic, computerized instruments for refraction have little practical application at present in rural eye clinics. The high initial purchase expense, the lack of maintenance, and the requirement of electric power make autorefractors impractical for widespread use in many countries.

Methods of measuring refractive error

Objective refraction with instruments

Streak retinoscopy

A trained refractionist can accurately determine the refractive state of the eye using the retinoscope by passing its beam of light (thc 'streak') across the pupil and noting the movement of the red reflex through lenses of varying strengths.
The light from the retinoscope is passed at different angles across the dilated pupil. The apparent motion of light reflected from the fundus is observed and 'neutralized' (brought to no apparent motion of light) by adding appropriate lenses. Streak retinoscopy can be learned from a skilled refractionist.

Autorefraction

Autorefraction is an accurate, objective method for determining refractive error.

Subjective refraction

The refractive error can be determined by testing vision with lenses of varying strength. Depending on the subjective response from the patient, appropriate lenses that provide best-corrected visual acuity can be determined. Many basic optical workshops do not produce cylindrical lenses. If cylindrical lenses are not available, appropriate spherical lenses can be provided.

Techniques for astigmatic refraction should be learned from an experienced refractionist. Caution should be observed in prescribing or providing cylindrical lenses for patients who have previously worn spherical lenses but have never worn cylindrical lenses, because of difficulty in adjusting to them.

Simplified myopic or hyperopic refraction

The following steps are suggested (not all steps may be necessary based on the clinical findings):

- Test the patient's vision separately in each eye with the pinhole. If vision is improved significantly by this, there is probably a refractive error.
- Refract the right eye first, and the left eye second, in the same order that ocular examination is performed.
- Begin by occluding the left eye. If using the trial frame, place the black occluder in the frame for the left eye.
- Place a +1.00 diopter lens in the trial frame in front of the right eye. If vision improves, assume that the patient is hyperopic. If vision is worse with the lens, assume that the patient is myopic.
- Remove the +1.00 diopter lens. (These instructions assume that the patient is found to be myopic. Reverse the sign of the following lenses if the patient is hyperopic.)
- Recheck the right eye with a series of minus lenses. Try minus lenses in −0.50 diopter intervals. (Check visual acuity with a −0.50 diopter lens first, then a −1.00 diopter lens, then a −1.50 diopter lens, and so on.)
- If vision improves with the addition of each −0.50 diopter lens, continue to add −0.50 diopter increments until vision no longer improves.
- Decrease the strength of the lens that gives best vision. To do so, gradually reduce the minus lens strength by −0.25 diopter decrements. The object is to provide only the minimum strength of minus lens necessary to give maximum vision. If too much minus lens power is prescribed, the patient will be 'over-minused' and the extra lens power will cause symptoms of 'pulling' or ocular discomfort.

■ Repeat the process for the left eye with the right eye occluded. Use the final prescription for the right eye as a guide for refracting the left eye because often the refractive error in both eyes is similar.

Simplified presbyopic refraction

The following steps are suggested (not all steps may be necessary based on the clinical findings):

■ When the patient complains of decreased near vision or difficulty reading, measure visual acuity of each eye separately, with and without glasses, at distance and at close range. Measure near visual acuity with a near visual acuity card (see inside front cover of this book) held at 40 cm (16 in). If the patient is wearing spectacles, determine the power of each lens with a lensometer.

■ If distance vision is 6/6 (20/20) or better in each eye without correction, assume that the patient is emmetropic.

■ Determine the patient's age and occupation. *Table 8* shows values which may be used as a guide for refraction.

■ Refract the right eye first and the left eye second. Try lenses in the ranges below according to the patient's age and visual requirements. For example, if spectacles are required for reading, check visual acuity with a near visual acuity card and trial lenses at the normal reading distance, usually about 40 cm (16 in).

■ Determine the least amount of plus lens power to give best vision at close range. Prescribing greater power in spectacle lenses for near vision will require the patient to hold reading material closer to the face. This will not significantly improve visual acuity and can inconvenience the patient.

■ Spectacles for near vision may be prescribed as single-vision spherical lenses. Inform patients who are using reading glasses for near work that their vision might be blurred with the same glasses for distance.

■ A simpler method of refracting presbyopes is to ask the patient to try reading with reading spectacles of various powers. The patient self-selects the spectacle power most suitable. Keep these trial spectacles with the examining equipment for this purpose.

Pseudophakic refraction

Patients who have undergone cataract surgery and have an IOL are left with no accommodation. They should be refracted according to their visual requirements.

The pseudophake may be able to read without reading glasses if the surgical result is slightly myopic (approximately 1 diopter). In such a case, distance refraction and correction are all that is necessary. The patient may remove glasses for reading. If the pseudophake is emmetropic after surgery, reading glasses will be necessary for reading and close work. If the patient is hyperopic after surgery, refraction and spectacle correction for both distance and close range will be necessary for clearest vision. Bifocals may be prescribed if they are available.

Table 8 Approximate requirements of presbyopes according to age

Age in years	Diopters
40 to 45	+1.25 to +1.50
45 to 50	+1.50 to +2.00
50 to 55	+2.00 to +2.50
55 to 60	+2.50 to +3.00

Aphakic refraction

Guidelines for aphakic refraction are as follows:

- All patients who have undergone cataract extraction should be optically corrected postoperatively (see Chapter 5).
- Most aphakic patients will require correction in the range of +10.00 to +12.00 diopters.
- Aphakic refraction may be performed by trial and error with lenses from the trial lens set or with aphakic spectacles of varying powers. The lenses that give best visual acuity at distance are prescribed.
- Maintaining a constant distance from the back surface of the aphakic lens to the patient's cornea is very important. Moving the spectacles forward or backward slightly will alter the patient's visual acuity. Aphakic spectacles should be fitted in the position at which visual acuity is best.
- For monocular aphakes (aphakia in one eye only) who have good vision in the other eye, vision in the aphakic eye should not be corrected with spectacles. Aphakic correction in one eye and normal or near-normal vision in the other eye results in image size differences and distortion (aniseikonia). A contact lens, if available, may be worn instead, if there is no contraindication. Extracapsular cataract extraction with IOL implantation can properly correct and balance vision when cataract surgery is indicated in only one eye.
- Aphakic spectacles can be prescribed for bilateral aphakes and for one-eyed patients who have had cataract surgery.
- Spherical aphakic spectacle lenses are less expensive and generally more widely available. Cylindrical aphakic lenses for astigmatic visual correction after cataract surgery are expensive and not widely available.

Asthenopia

Asthenopia is the technical term for eye strain, or discomfort with prolonged use. It is one of the most common complaints from patients, particularly school children, in eye clinics. Asthenopia is not damaging to the eyes; it is only uncomfortable. A complete ocular examination should be performed to check for possible ocular disease. If no disease is present, visual acuity is normal, and the patient is emmetropic or nearly so, no medications should be given. Asthenopia is common in the following situations:

- After reading (headache, aching of eyes, and tearing with reading are all symptoms of asthenopia).
- In students, particularly near examination time when students increase their reading and studying.
- In individuals with mild hyperopia, because they must constantly accommodate to see clearly.

The problem should be explained to the patient and advice offered about how to reduce symptoms from asthenopia. Appropriate advice includes the following:

- These symptoms are not damaging to the eyes and it is safe to continue to read.
- To minimize glare, the light source should be from behind or beside the reader rather than from in front.
- Hold reading material a suitable distance from the eyes. The closer the reading material, the more accommodation must be exerted to see properly and the greater the asthenopic symptoms.
- At the first indication of ocular discomfort, the reader should rest and discontinue reading for a few minutes until the discomfort disappears.

Special considerations

Spectacles are readily available in wealthy nations where resources are abundant and demand is high. Even small refractive errors are often corrected with eyeglasses, and prescription sunglasses are prescribed for photophobia. Eyeglasses are worn sometimes only for fashion.

In countries where government and private resources are limited, spectacles are worn by only a small proportion of the people who need them. Most people with refractive errors go uncorrected.

For those people who cannot afford to purchase commercially produced spectacles, low-cost spherical optical correction can be provided. A national program for the prevention of blindness should include provision of low-cost spectacles to patients with aphakia, myopia, and presbyopia (**155**).

Low-cost optical workshops can produce spectacles from optical scrap and other inexpensive materials. Such workshops often employ disabled individuals as opticians and technicians in rehabilitation projects. High-quality spectacles with spherical corrections of standard powers are also produced commercially in quantity in several countries and sold at reasonable cost.

Service clubs, including Lions Clubs and Rotary Clubs, collect unused and second-hand spectacles for donation and free distribution to indigent patients. The power of the lenses can be determined with a lensometer. Spectacles are then prescribed for patients who have undergone examination and refraction. Donated spectacles with spherical lenses (not cylindrical lenses) are the most valuable for this purpose.

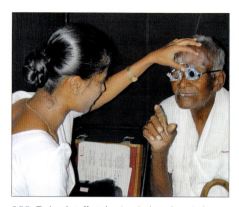

155 Trained staff at the Aravind eye hospitals, India, refract the referred patients, note down their refractive error and write out the prescription.

14

Low vision

People need to know what constitutes the difference between normal vision and impairment, the potential benefits of low-vision care, and where to go for services.
World Health Organization low-vision workshop, Madrid, 1996

Project Vision 2020 aims to eliminate the major causes of blindness by bringing together governments and non-governmental organizations to facilitate the development, planning, and implementation of sustainable eye care programmes.
IAPB and WHO

There are more than three times as many people with low vision as there are people who are blind. Approximately 90% of blindness and low vision occurs in the developing world and approximately 80% of blindness is "avoidable," that is, it can be prevented or corrected. Please see Appendix F for definitions of blindness and low vision.

Low vision services should be integrated into all eye care programmes. Awareness, recognition and correction of low vision should be promoted among eye care workers, public service organizations working for prevention of blindness, and health agencies. In addition to refraction, and cataract surgery when appropriate, there are simple interventions that can assist people with low vision and significantly improve their eyesight and their lives. Basic optical workshops can also produce simple low-vision optical devices at modest cost. See appendix G for a list of organizations that can provide further information on low vision services.

Table 9 **Global estimate of blindness and low vision***	
Total number visually impaired (blind and low vision)	161 million
Total blind	37 million
Total low vision	124 million
Blind chlldren	1.4 million
* All data: WHO 2004	

Definitions

Visual acuity is a measurement of the eye's capacity to see detail (sharpness of vision, dependent on the macula of the retina). Distance visual acuity is a measurement of the ability to read standard figures on a chart at 6 m (20 ft). *Near visual acuity* is a measurement of the ability to read standard figures on a card at 40 cm (16 in). *Vision* is the sense of sight as a whole, which includes visual acuity and peripheral, or side, vision (visual field). (The term vision is not equivalent to visual acuity.) *Functional vision* is visual acuity and peripheral vision sufficient for the person to carry out his or her normal activities.

Low vision, or *functional visual impairment*, is a significant limitation of visual capability resulting from disease, trauma, or congenital condition that cannot be corrected to the normal range with refraction, medical treatment, or surgery. Such impairment may be manifested by insufficient visual resolution, inadequate field of vision, or reduced peak contrast sensitivity. Even after therapeutic measures are taken, the patient may still remain with visual impairment or low vision. The formal World Health Organization definition of low vision is a visual acuity of less than 6/18 (20/60) and equal to or better than 3/60 (20/400) in the better eye (see Appendix F). A person who has better than 6/18 visual acuity in the better eye, but peripheral vision of less than 10°, also has low vision.

Causes of low vision

There are numerous causes of low vision. A large percentage of people with impaired vision can be helped.

Cataract

Cataract which is not surgically treated is the single most common cause of blindness and low vision in the world.

Refractive error

Uncorrected high refractive errors – high myopia of more than – 6.00 diopters or high hyperopia of more than +3.00 diopters – are common causes of low vision. Precise data on refractive errors as a cause of low vision on a global scale are not available. It is very important to refract all people with low vision. Visual acuity can often be improved, although not always to normal visual acuity.

Corneal scarring

An irregular corneal surface from xerophthalmia (due to vitamin A deficiency), corneal ulcer, or injury can produce mild scarring (nebulae), distortion of vision, and low vision. More severe corneal scarring (maculae and leucomata) from trachoma and other causes is common in many regions with inadequate eye care and is a major cause of low vision. Corneal grafting (transplantation) is impractical for corneal scarring from trachoma because of poor surgical results.

Macular degeneration

Degeneration of the macula is most commonly related to aging (age-related macular degeneration) and is usually bilateral. This is a more serious problem in countries where life expectancy is high and a large percentage of the population is elderly. Inherited macular degeneration may also occur in young adults, but it is less common. Macular degeneration will become an increasing problem in the developing world in the coming decades as populations in economically developing countries become greater and life expectancy rises.

Glaucoma

Both angle-closure glaucoma and open-angle glaucoma may be responsible for low vision. Peripheral vision (used for moving about and finding things in the larger environment) is usually lost initially in glaucoma. Because visual acuity (central macular vision, used for reading and detail work) may be good until late in the disease course, a person with glaucoma (particularly open-angle glaucoma) may not even be aware that the disease is present until central visual acuity is affected. When central acuity is affected in glaucoma, there is usually severe peripheral vision loss present also.

Ocular trauma

Ocular trauma, including surface injuries and penetrating intraocular injuries, may cause low vision.

Onchocerciasis

Secondary uveitis, corneal scarring, and glaucoma from onchocerciasis is a major cause of low vision in western and central African nations.

Diabetic retinopathy

Diabetic retinopathy, a retinal vascular complication of diabetes mellitus, is a common cause of low vision in industrialized countries. At present, diabetic retinopathy is not a common condition in most developing nations, but it will become more common as insulin and other treatments become more available and diabetic patients live longer.

Congenital causes

Low vision may be due to inherited congenital causes. An infant or child with a congenital visual defect should be treated as soon as possible after diagnosis and referred for special educational assistance.

Retinopathy of prematurity

Premature infants subjected to high oxygen levels in incubators may develop neovascularization of the retina, resulting in extensive damage to the retina, macula, vitreous, and lens. It is usually bilateral, and the visual acuity may be severely affected.

Professional, patient, and public awareness

Professional eye care workers are often unaware of the possibilities for detecting usable vision in their patients with low vision and for providing assistance that will allow them to function more effectively. All too often, a patient with a degenerative disease or an inoperable condition and low vision is not evaluated properly by medical and non-medical eye care practitioners. If low vision cannot be improved by an accurate refraction or by cataract surgery, the patient should be considered for fitting with a low-vision aid. Proper referral should be made by eye health care practitioners to low-vision services, non-governmental organizations, and societies for the vision impaired.

Patients should be informed that they can be helped by a low-vision professional if their vision is impaired but cannot be improved by surgery or refraction. Patients should be referred to an eye health care worker experienced in low vision examination and treatment.

Public health information and educational materials on low vision should be included in comprehensive national, regional, and local blindness prevention and sight restoration programs. Organizations working with blindness prevention and cataract programs should also refer people with low vision for further evaluation and treatment. Community leaders should know the value of screening for low vision and blindness, and should be encouraged to support these programs.

Low-vision care

Identification and screening

To determine the extent of vision loss, visual acuity should be measured, first testing both eyes together and then testing each eye separately. Accurate visual acuity measurements in each eye – together with the eye examination – are necessary to determine if low vision is present and how it may be helped. (If standard visual acuity charts are in scarce supply, they can be reproduced by local printers; see Chapter 3.)

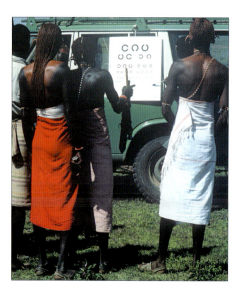

Visual acuity should be measured in each eye at distance (6 m, or 20 ft) without spectacles and then with spectacles if the person wears them. First check the right eye, then the left eye. Then check each eye with the pinhole. Pinhole testing can help identify whether the patient's visual acuity can be improved with refraction and prescription of glasses. Poor visual acuity from certain types of cataract (especially posterior subcapsular cataract) may also be improved with the pinhole test.

Visual acuity should also be measured at near using a standard near card (see inside front cover of this book). Each eye should be measured separately; check the right eye first, followed by the left eye. If the patient is literate and a near reading card is not available, use small newspaper type for this test.

If the person is not literate, the E optotypes (visual acuity test objects) should be used. The E optotypes – individual or pointed out on a chart – are usually used at 6 m (20 ft) and are rotated in the four directions in a random sequence. The patient identifies the direction the E is facing. Smaller E optotypes for near visual acuity are read at the distance the person is accustomed to holding printed material. The E may be described as a 'rake' or a 'hoe' if the person does not understand the letter designation. This comparison may be useful in agricultural societies.

Other optotypes, such as a C figure, may also be used. The person whose visual acuity is being measured points in the direction of the opening in the circle. The Landolt ring (C) optotype may be likened to an enclosure and the opening to its door. This comparison may better suit nomads who are not literate but who keep cattle in an enclosure (156).

156 Testing visual acuity in the field with a Landolt ring (C) visual acuity chart in a nomadic population.

Performing low-vision testing

Face the patient. Demonstrate how to do the E test by showing how to indicate the direction the Es (or Cs) point. Test distance and near vision to find the smallest character the patient can see.

Distance vision. Test the person both with spectacles if they are normally used for distance tasks and without. Count how many optotypes are identified correctly, in the following sequence:

1 Test with the four small Es at 6 m (20 ft).

- Vision is normal (6/18 [20/60] or better) if at least three out of four small Es can be seen.

- If the patient is not able to see at least three of the small Es, go to step 2.

2 Test with the large E at 6 m. Turn the card to test the E in four different (random) directions.

- If at least three of four Es are identified correctly, vision is at least 6/60 (20/200). Low vision is moderate (6/18–6/60). Check the pinhole vision; if improved, test for improvement with spectacles; if not improved, refer to eye specialist.

- If the patient is not able to see at least three of the large Es, go to step 3.

3 Test with the large E at 3 m (10 feet). Turn the card to test the E in four different (random) directions.

- If at least three of four Es are identified correctly, visual acuity is at least 3/60 (20/400). Low vision is severe (6/60–3/60). Repeat the pinhole test to see if vision is improved.

- If the patient is not able to identify at least three of the large Es, test with the pinhole and refer to an eye specialist for possible treatment. Low vision is profound (<3/60).

Near vision. Let the person hold the near vision optotypes as close as desired. Test from the largest to the smallest Es. At least three out of four must be correct in each line before testing the next. If only the largest size can be seen, check if magnifiers will help and test for spectacles; refer to an eye specialist for possible treatment. The medium size is similar to the print in large-print books. The smallest size is similar to print in books and magazines.

Note: If the near vision optotypes are used at 6 m and the largest Es can be correctly identified, the patient's vision is 6/6 (20/20).

General doctors or community health care workers can be a valuable resource for identifying people with low vision. With proper training, religious groups, clubs, and community groups can also screen people for low vision and provide them with referrals and information on eye care.

The algorithm above is designed specifically for use with the World Health Organization/University of Melbourne low-vision optotypes. A more general algorithm for measuring visual acuity with a standard Snellen chart and counting fingers is given in Chapter 16. Chapter 13 describes the basics of trial lens refraction.

Appropriate lighting and glare reduction

For reading, low light (dim illumination) does not bring out contrast in the printed matter well. A brighter light source (higher illumination) will produce greater contrast between the background (paper) and the target (printed numbers or letters) and make reading easier. A low-intensity light source may be placed closer to reading material for greater contrast if brighter artificial light is not available.

The position of the light source for reading is very important. The light should be placed in a position that will not produce glare for the reader. Glare is overly bright light or reflection from a smooth surface that interferes with vision. Glare can further increase reading problems of people with low vision. To prevent glare, the light source can be positioned behind the reader or obliquely from the side so that light does not reflect directly off the page into the reader's eyes. Bright light from an overhead source may be decreased by having the patient wear a hat with a brim while reading. Tinted spectacle lenses may also reduce glare, create greater contrast, and make reading easier.

If artificial light is not available, natural light is necessary for reading. Reading material should be positioned to avoid glare, increase contrast, and avoid shadows on the printed page to realize maximum benefit.

Optical aids: low-vision devices
Spectacles
Presbyopic people who wear spectacles for distance require a second lens for reading because of loss of accommodation. Bifocal lenses are usually prescribed for this purpose.

A +3.00 diopter bifocal add is usually the maximum effective power for near vision in a normally sighted individual who is more than 60 years of age or a high hyperope. Single-vision spectacles of greater than +3.00 diopters (6- to 10-diopter magnifying glasses) may be helpful for people with low vision. Reading matter must be held closer to the face to be seen with high-plus spectacles.

Hand-held magnifying lenses
The patient may find a hand-held magnifying lens more convenient than magnifying spectacles. Generally, the larger the area of the magnifying glass, the easier it is for the patient to read the magnified type.

(Magnification usually decreases with broader [wider] hand lenses. Larger lenses usually magnify less but offer wider fields of view.) This increased ease of reading occurs because of the larger field resulting from the larger area of glass. Such a large field is more helpful to a patient with severe low vision than a small magnifying lens. For patients with low vision who are only minimally affected by their disease, a small pocket magnifier may be useful for reading the smallest type.

Telescopes
Small telescopes that fit on spectacle lenses may be helpful and convenient for some people with low vision who require improved vision. Most telescopes are hand-held, however, and are difficult to use because of their small field of view. Telescopes are more expensive than hand-held magnifiers and magnifying spectacles and are difficult to fit properly on spectacles. Because of their expense, their usefulness for most people with low vision in developing nations is limited.

Non-optical aids
Many of the low vision devices (LVDs) available in industrialized countries are too expensive to be practical for developing countries at present and are not widely available. Not only are these devices expensive, but they may require maintenance which is not available. Such LVDs include talking machines, scanning machines that read aloud, and television monitor screens that display magnified images. Practical non-optical aids are large-print books, newspapers, and magazines. Enlarging printed numbers, figures, and words acts to magnify the reading material. Many literate people with low vision find such printed material helpful.

Part 3

Ophthalmology backgrounder

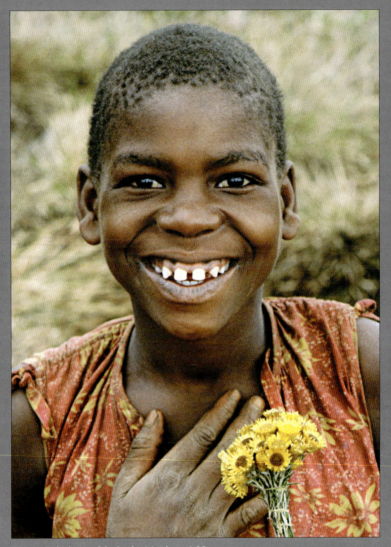

The eye is the lamp of the body : Matthew 6:22

15

Anatomy and physiology

Fearfully and wonderfully made
Psalms 139:14

A basic understanding of the anatomical features and normal function of the human eye is necessary before potentially blinding diseases can be recognized and treated. The information presented in this chapter is basic and introductory; it is neither detailed nor comprehensive. Students may learn the fundamentals of anatomy and physiology from this chapter, but for more thorough study of the form and function of the human visual system, a standard textbook of ophthalmology should be consulted.

Anatomy of the human eye and adnexa

This discussion begins with the external anatomical landmarks and is followed by the anatomy of the eyeball from its external to its internal features. The text then describes the various parts of the adnexa, proceeding from external through internal anatomy. There is no best order of discussion, because the visual system is an integrated, linked whole, and each aspect involves discussion of other anatomical features.

General external anatomy and landmarks

The eyebrow marks the upper extent of the upper eyelid and overlies the bony orbital rim. Because it extends beyond the anterior plane of the eye, the bony rim of the orbit provides protection for the eye from injury.

The upper and lower eyelids also protect and shield the eye. The lateral canthus is the junction of the eyelids laterally and the medial canthus is the junction of the eyelids medially.

A tough, strong tissue, the sclera, gives the white color to a healthy eye. The conjunctiva overlies the sclera and the inner surfaces of the eyelids. A healthy conjunctiva is transparent, but sometimes small normal blood vessels may be seen.

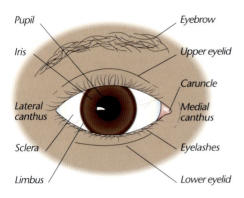

157 External anatomy of the eye.

The small mound of conjunctiva in the medial canthus is the caruncle. The iris and pupil are visible through the cornea, the transparent window at the front of the eye. The limbus forms the boundary between the clear cornea and the opaque sclera (**157**).

External anatomy of the eyeball

Measuring approximately 2.5 cm in diameter, the normal adult eyeball is almost spherical. Its volume is about 7 ml. The eyeball is positioned in the bony orbit and is supported in its position by Tenon's capsule, a connective tissue similar to muscle fascia that surrounds the posterior eyeball and extends anteriorly to the conjunctival fornix between the conjunctiva and sclera.

The cornea is the anterior surface of the anterior chamber. The normal cornea is 10.5–12 mm in diameter and approximately 1 mm thick. It is composed of five distinct layers. These layers, from the external surface to the internal surface of the cornea, are epithelium, Bowman's membrane, stroma, Descemet's membrane, and endothelium (**158**).

The sclera, which is also about 1 mm in thickness, is the firm white external supporting tissue of the eyeball. The optic nerve, which transmits visual signals from the retina to the area of the brain where vision is interpreted, attaches to the posterior pole of the eyeball at the sclera.

The conjunctiva overlies Tenon's capsule and sclera and inserts at the limbus. The conjunctiva overlying the anterior surface of the eyeball (bulbar conjunctiva) is continuous with the tarsal conjunctiva, which forms the posterior surface of the eyelids. The eyelid recesses are the upper (superior) and lower (inferior) fornices.

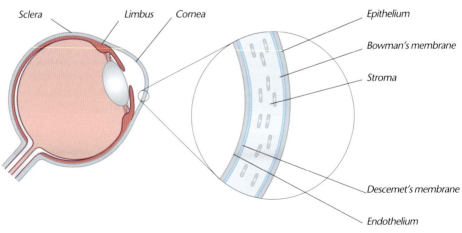

158 Layers of the cornea.

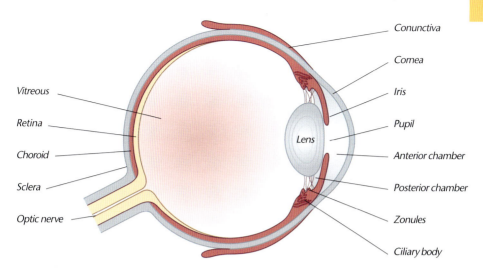

159 Cross-section of the external and internal anatomy of the human eye.

Internal anatomy of the eyeball

The eyeball as a whole (**159**) is often referred to as the globe. The space lying between the endothelium of the cornea and the iris is the anterior chamber. The anterior chamber contains aqueous fluid which is constantly being produced by the ciliary body and which drains out of the eyeball through a microscopic ring of porous tissue called the trabecular meshwork located at the periphery of the anterior chamber just anterior to the iris. Taken together, the base of the iris, the trabecular meshwork, and supporting scleral and corneal tissue are known as the angle (**160**). The circular opening in the iris is the pupil.

Posterior to the iris is the crystalline lens. (See Figure 38 for a drawing of the structure of the lens.) It is suspended in position by the zonules (zonular ligament), which are attached to the ciliary processes of the ciliary body. The space peripheral to the lens and just posterior to the iris is called the posterior chamber. (Note that the posterior chamber is not the space in which the vitreous is situated.)

The vitreous (vitreous body) is the largest tissue of the eyeball. It occupies the vitreous cavity, the space bounded by the posterior lens, zonules, ciliary body, and retina. Vitreous is a clear, jellylike tissue that becomes more fluid with age.

Three distinct anatomical structures compose the uvea, or uveal tract: iris; ciliary body; and choroid. Although the three components of the uveal tract are

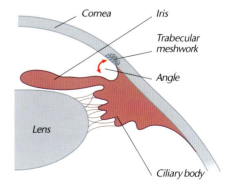

160 Structures of the angle: iris, trabecular meshwork, and cornea.

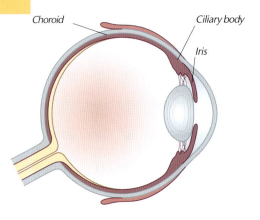

161 Structures of the uveal tract: iris, ciliary body, and choroid.

attached to each other, making the uvea a continuous tissue, each structure has a distinct and separate function. The iris serves to regulate light entering the eye through the space in its center, the pupil. The ciliary body supports the zonules, produces aqueous, and its small muscles are active in accommodation (see Chapter 13 for explanation of accommodation). The choroid is a vascular tissue positioned between the retina and sclera (**161**).

The retina, a delicate neurosensory tissue composed of 10 microscopic layers, is the innermost layer lining the back of the eyeball. Millions of microscopic cone cells, which are sensitive to bright light, and rod cells, which are sensitive to dim light, are located in the retina. Cones and rods are known as photoreceptors. The greatest density of photoreceptors is in the macula, the slightly depressed dark spot near the center of the retina (**162**). There are approximately 1 million cones in a healthy human macula.

The photoreceptors transform energy from light into tiny currents of electrical energy, which are transmitted to the brain through the visual pathway by means of the optic nerve. The retina and the optic nerve are nervous tissue extensions of the brain in the eye.

The insertion of the optic nerve into the sclera and its attachment to retinal fibers is medial (nasal) to the macula. When performing funduscopy with the ophthalmoscope, the observer visualizes the optic nerve head (optic disc) as being either to the left or the right of the macula, depending on the eye being examined. The optic cup is the normal depression in the center of the optic nerve. The arteries and veins serving the retina enter the eye through the optic cup.

The cornea, anterior chamber, iris, trabecular meshwork, supporting sclera, and lens, considered together, are known as the anterior segment. The ciliary body, choroid, vitreous, retina, optic nerve head (optic disc), and supporting sclera, taken together, are known as the posterior segment. A rich network of blood vessels serves the external and internal eyeball and the optic nerve.

Optic nerve and visual system

The length of the optic nerve from its connection at the sclera to the optic canal is about 2.5 cm. The optic nerve is composed of millions tiny nerve fibers. After leaving the optic canal at the far posterior aspect of the orbit, the optic nerve meets and crosses the optic nerve from the opposite eye at the optic chiasm.

Nerve fibers of the optic nerve connect with other neurons (nervous system cells), which end in the occipital cortex in the posterior part of the brain. There the neural signals that were originally converted from light energy by photoreceptors of the retina are interpreted as visual images in color.

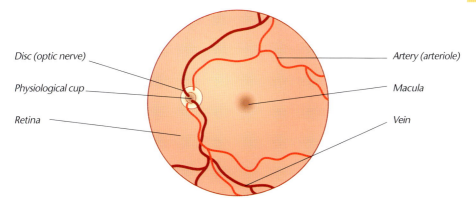

162 Normal retina, optic disc, normal (physiological) cup, blood vessels, and macula of left eye, as viewed by direct ophthalmoscopy.

Eyelids

The eyelid is composed of four basic layers. From the external surface to the internal surface, these layers are skin, muscle, tarsal plate, and conjunctiva (**163**).

The orbicularis oculi muscle, responsible for eyelid closure, is the major muscle of the eyelids. There are two additional muscles in the upper eyelid, the levator muscle and Müller's muscle. The levator muscle elevates the upper eyelid. Müller's muscle provides support and also helps to elevate the upper eyelid.

Normal eyelids contain fat glands, mucus glands, and small lacrimal (tear) glands, all of which contribute secretions to the tear film. Most of the eyelid glands are situated on the upper and lower eyelid margins. The tear film provides constant lubrication and moisture for the ocular surface, which are essential for a healthy eye. Eyelashes (cilia), also located on the eyelid margins, provide protection for the eye from small foreign bodies.

The tarsus (tarsal plate), a firm, fibrous tissue, provides form and stability to the eyelids, especially the upper eyelid. It is very important to know the anatomy of the tarsus and to understand its function in

order to perform entropion (trichiasis) surgery to correct eyelid deformities from chronic trachoma (see Chapter 7). The tarsus of the lower eyelid is thinner and shorter than the tarsus of the upper eyelid. The fornices (eyelid recesses) are covered by a continuous layer of conjunctiva.

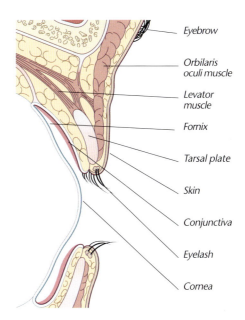

163 Anatomy of the eyelid.

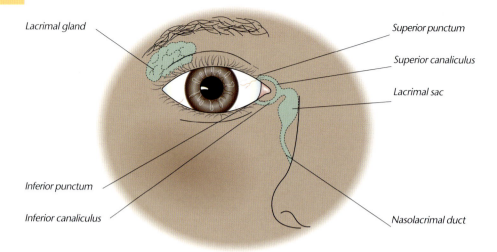

Lacrimal gland

Superior punctum

Superior canaliculus

Lacrimal sac

Inferior punctum

Inferior canaliculus

Nasolacrimal duct

164 The lacrimal system.

Lacrimal system

The lacrimal gland is situated in the anterior superior temporal orbit beneath the eyelid. A healthy lacrimal gland produces tears that drain from the gland through numerous tiny ducts into the superior temporal fornix. The tears form a thin fluid layer (the tear film) over the epithelial surface of the cornea and conjunctiva. Tears provide moisture and lubrication.

The tears drain away from the eye into the lacrimal sac through the lacrimal canaliculi. Each canaliculus opens onto the eyelid. The opening is known as the punctum. One punctum is positioned on each eyelid near the medial canthus. Tears drain from the lacrimal sac into the nose through the nasolacrimal duct (**164**).

Extraocular muscles

There are three pairs of extraocular muscles that attach to and move the eyeball: two horizontal muscles, the lateral rectus and medial rectus; two vertical muscles, the superior rectus and inferior rectus; and two oblique muscles, the superior oblique and inferior oblique.

These six muscles originate from within the orbit and each attaches to the eyeball at the sclera. Each extraocular muscle has specific and independent functions in moving the eyeball and corresponds to a specific muscle in the fellow eye to move both eyes together in the same direction.

Bony orbit

The bony orbit, the space that holds the eyeball and all supporting structures, is composed of parts of seven bones. It is approximately the shape of a cone (the posterior aspect is the apex) and is approximately 30 ml in volume. The superior, inferior, medial, and lateral orbital rims form the anterior edges of the orbit. The optic nerve, other cranial nerves and blood vessels that serve the eyeball, the extraocular muscles, and the eyelids pass through openings near the orbital apex into the cranial cavity. A thin but firm orbital septum, attached to the orbital rim and the eyelids, protects the delicate orbital structures from external penetrating injuries and infections.

Physiology of the human eye

The eye is a sensitive sensory organ. The visual system – eyes, support structures, and neurosensory brain connections – makes possible the sense of sight, perhaps the most important of human senses. To work effectively, the eye depends on proper functioning of many systems, especially nerves, blood supply, muscles, fluids, and the optic pathway to the brain.

General considerations

Both eyes together, if correctly aligned, see the same image simultaneously. Extra-ocular muscles cause the eyes to track together, yielding a binocular image in the brain. Binocular vision makes it possible to judge spaces between objects (depth perception).

The normal cornea is clear and transparent; it has no blood vessels. Corneal nutrition is provided through aqueous fluid and tear film. An optically clear cornea is essential for good vision. The clear structures of the eye – tear film, cornea, aqueous, lens, and vitreous – are known as the ocular media and provide a clear, un-interrupted pathway for light to reach the retina. An opacity in the media (such as a corneal scar or a lens opacity) will cause loss of vision. An adequate tear film is essential for a healthy eye; without the tear film, the cornea loses its clarity and the conjunctiva dries.

The iris serves as a diaphragm and thus controls the amount of light entering the eye. By expanding and contracting, the iris regulates the size of the pupil. If the light source is bright, the pupil contracts to allow less light to reach the retina. In dim light or darker conditions, the pupil enlarges to allow more light into the eye.

The ciliary body contains muscle tissue and is capable of changing its shape by contraction and relaxation of these muscles. Ciliary body muscular contraction and relaxation cause thickening and thinning of the lens and allow the lens to change the focus of light on the retina. This process is known as accommodation.

The crystalline lens continues to enlarge slightly throughout life; the lens in the eye of a newborn is smaller than an adult lens. The epithelium under the anterior capsule continues to produce new lens cells; not only does this cause the lens to enlarge, but it becomes firmer with age. Hardening of the lens with age decreases its ability to accommodate, causing presbyopia (loss of visual acuity at close range due to loss of accommodation). This condition normally begins at approximately age 40 years in a person without a refractive error.

The third part of the uveal system, the choroid, is a layer of highly vascularized tissue between the sclera and the retina in the posterior eyeball. Its function is to nourish the retina through its small-blood-vessel network, and to support the retina's role in the rapid transmission of electrical signals to the brain.

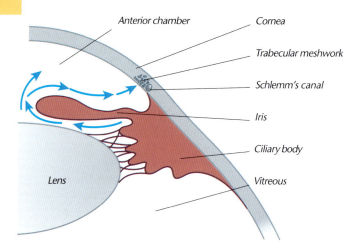

165 Normal path of aqueous through the eye.

Aqueous fluid

Aqueous is constantly being formed in the epithelium of the ciliary body and is secreted into the posterior chamber (**165**). From the posterior chamber, aqueous passes through the pupil into the anterior chamber. It then passes out of the anterior chamber through the trabecular meshwork into Schlemm's canal and from there, by tiny channels, out of the eyeball into vessels of the conjunctiva.

The steady creation and drainage of aqueous fluid maintain a particular intraocular pressure (IOP), or firmness, within the eye. Normal IOP of the human eye is 10–21 mmHg. If aqueous is created faster than it is drained, IOP is elevated and the pathological processes of glaucoma may result (see Chapter 6).

16

The eye examination

Where observation is concerned, chance favors only the prepared mind.
Louis Pasteur

A good ocular history and examination are essential to establishing a correct diagnosis. Learning a few key skills will enable the student of ophthalmology to identify most ocular diseases in simple settings using uncomplicated equipment. This chapter describes the basic eye examination. Instruction from an experienced eye health care worker and continuous practice are necessary to fully master these techniques.

General considerations

Train your powers of observation. A good examiner always pays attention to details. Consider the many possible diagnoses, both ocular and systemic, when examining eye patients.

Keep accurate history, examination, and treatment records. In some health care outpatient facilities, patients keep in their possession their own records. Notes written on those outpatient records should be just as accurate and concise as those written in hospital records for inpatients.

Hands and fingernails should be clean at all times when examining eye patients. Wash your hands after examination of any patient with an eye infection. Surgical spirits and cotton wool can be used to clean hands quickly when screening many patients and especially for examining post-operative patient‚s who require meticulous sterile care.

Always examine the right eye first and the left eye second even if the patient complains of a problem only in the left eye. This routine ensures that an examination of both eyes has been performed and lessens the possibility that an abnormality in the right eye is overlooked.

The ocular history

Listen carefully to the patient's history and record it accurately and concisely. Record age, sex, and occupation of the patient. Determine the length of time the eye complaint has been present. Time of occurrence is especially important for ocular injuries as well as how the injury happened.

If the patient has already been treated for an eye complaint, note the medications the patient is using or has used. In particular, ask about the use of corticosteroid drops or ointment, antibiotic use, and glaucoma medications. If a traditional herbal, animal, or non-therapeutic chemical medication has been used or the patient has been treated by a traditional healer with any of those substances or by mechanical or thermal manipulation, that information should also be recorded in the ocular history.

The ocular examination

A complete ophthalmic examination includes the following elements:

- Visual acuity measurement.
- Pinhole tessting in any eye with subnormal vision.
- Refraction if necessary
- Cross-confrontation visual-field testing (see Chapter 6).
- Motility (movement) and binocular alignment testing (integrity of the extraocular muscles).
- External examination, including eyelids, sclera, cornea, conjunctiva, and lacrimal system.
- Anterior segment examination, including anterior chamber depth, pupillary reactivity and size, and status of the lens (possible presence of cataract).
- Possible presence of opacity of the media.
- Posterior segment examination of the fundus of the eye, including the retina, macula, and optic nerve.
- Tonometry (measurement of intra-ocular pressure)

These elements of the exam need not be done in this specific order, although visual acuity testing is usually performed first. As inspection of the ocular media and the posterior segment requires dilation of the pupil with a mydriatic drop (causing blurred vision), inspection of the internal structures of the eye is usually done last.

Visual acuity

The single most important measurement in the ocular examination is visual acuity. Every patient should undergo visual acuity measurements in both eyes. The results are then recorded in the health care record. An accurate visual acuity can be taken using standard figures or optotypes. The Snellen chart consists of letters or numbers printed in decreasing sizes according to an international standard. (If standard visual acuity charts are in scarce supply, they can be reproduced by local printers; see Chapter 3.) The notations on the Snellen visual acuity chart may be in meters or in feet. The 'normal' visual acuity is 6/6 (meters) or 20/20 (feet).

Common abbreviations used for recording visual acuity include the following:

- V (vision).
- RE (right eye) or OD (oculus dexter).
- LE (left eye) or OS (oculus sinister).
- NV (near vision).
- PH (pinhole).
- CF (count fingers).
- NLP (no light perception).

A general algorithm for measuring visual acuity using the Snellen chart and finger counting is given opposite (the exact sequence of testing may vary based on specific circumstances). Measure the right eye first, record the result, then measure the left eye and record the result. A specific algorithm for use with low-vision opto-types is given in Chapter 14. If refractive error is found, see Chapter 13 for methods of refractive testing and correction.

Measuring visual acuity

1 Position the patient 6 m (20 ft) from the Snellen chart.

2 Explain the test to the patient and direct the patient's attention to the Snellen chart.

3 Ask the patient to cover the left eye to test the right eye first. The examiner may cover the patient's left eye with an opaque shield rather than the hand. Observe the patient closely as the test proceeds because patients sometimes will attempt to look at the chart by peeking from behind the shield if the eye being tested does not have normal vision.

4 Ask the patient to read line by line down the chart until the smallest line is reached that the patient can read accurately. Record the testing distance first (6 m), a slash (/), then the smallest line read second. For example, if the patient read most or all of the 18 line on the metric chart, then visual acuity would be recorded '6/18'; if the Snellen chart is measured in feet and the patient read the 60 line, then the visual acuity would be recorded '20/60.'

5 If the patient is not literate, use an E chart or Landolt ring C chart (see Figure 11) and ask the patient to indicate the direction the figures are facing.

6 The patient's vision may be so poor that figures on the chart cannot be read. In this case, direct the patient's attention to the outstretched fingers on your hand and ask the patient to count the number of fingers you are holding up at various distances. Record the best finger-counting vision. If fingers are counted correctly at 5 m, for example, record the visual acuity as 'counts fingers 5 m.' (Because the fingers are similar in size to the 60 size E at the top of the chart, this visual acuity may also be written '5/60.' If the patient can only count fingers at 3 m, then the visual acuity is '3/60,' and so on.)

7 If the patient cannot count fingers at close range, then determine if focal light from a flashlight (torch) can be seen in each of four retinal quadrants. To do this, hold the light 10 cm from the eye, just in front of the face and pointing in toward the eye, in positions of up and out (superotemporal); up and in (superonasal); down and out (inferotemporal); and down and in (inferonasal); and ask the patient to point to the direction of the light. If the patient correctly points to the source of the light in each case, he or she is able to project light and the visual acuity is recorded as 'accurate light projection.' If the patient makes a mistake in one or more quadrants, then the visual acuity is 'inaccurate light projection.'

8 If light from the flashlight cannot be seen at all, then vision is recorded as 'no light perception' or 'NLP.' It is not appropriate to record 'blind' as a visual measurement on a medical record because the word blind has a negative connotation in many societies.

If the patient's visual acuity is less than 6/6 (20/20) in one or both eyes, then attempt to measure visual acuity through a pinhole. A pinhole device is contained in the trial lens set for refraction; if a trial lens set is unavailable, a small pinhole can be created from X-ray film or cardboard (see Chapter 3). Record the vision as 'PH 6/9,' for example, if the patient reads that line. If visual acuity is improved with the pinhole test, then refractive error, especially myopia (nearsightedness), is a likely etiology for decreased visual acuity and a refraction should be performed.

If the patient complains of poor near vision or is 40 years of age or older, then check near visual acuity at a distance of 40 cm (16 in) with a standard near visual acuity chart (see inside front cover of this book). Each eye should be tested separately and the result recorded in the health care record.

External ocular examination

Inspection of the eyelids and the external eye can be performed with two simple instruments: a good focal flashlight (torch) and a binocular loupe or hand magnifying glass. A slit lamp (biomicroscope), if available, is very useful but not essential to perform an adequate examination (see also Cnapter 3, Figure 13).

Carefully examine the eyelid surfaces and margins with the flashlight and magnifying lens. Note any abnormality.

Check for normal muscle motility (movement) by having the patient look in the six cardinal fields of gaze (right and up, right, right and down, left and up, left, left and down). Check for binocular alignment with the corneal reflex test. To do a corneal reflex test, ask the patient to fixate straight ahead (primary position) on the vision chart at 6 m and direct the flashlight from straight ahead into the center of the patient's face from a distance of 20 cm. A light reflex should be centered on each cornea (in the center of the pupil). If the light reflections are not both centered, the patient may have strabismus (see Chapter 12 and Figure 151). If the light reflex is temporal (lateral) to the corneal center, the condition is probably esotropia. If the light reflex is nasal (medial) to the corneal center, the condition is probably exotropia. If the light reflex is superior or inferior, the diagnosis is probably hypertropia.

Note any scar or abnormality of the cornea. Corneal scarring is classified as follows:

- Leukoma – white opaque scar.
- Macula – translucent spot (admits or transmits some light); do not confuse the term corneal macula with the macula of the retina.
- Nebula – mild superficial scar that is difficult to see without magnification.

Examine the sclera and the bulbar and tarsal conjunctiva with the flashlight and magnifier. The upper eyelid must be everted in order to examine the tarsal conjunctiva. To evert the eyelid, grasp the eyelashes with the fingers of one hand and turn the tarsal plate up over a matchstick or a clean fingertip of the other hand (**166**).

If the patient complains of tearing, carefully examine all four puncta and attempt to gently express any material that may be in the lacrimal sacs back through the inferior puncta. If pus or mucus is expressed, then there is probably a blockage in the lacrimal drainage system.

Fluorescein stain is useful for identifying a defect in the corneal or conjunctival epithelium. (*Pseudomonas* bacteria can grow easily in moist environments, particularly fluorescein, and fluorescein drops contaminated with *Pseudomonas* can cause serious ocular infection; hence it is

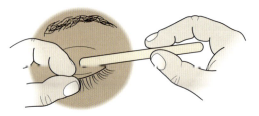
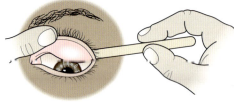

a   b

166 Eversion of the upper eyelid: ask patient to look down; grasp upper eyelashes with thumb and forefinger (a); turn upper eyelid up over matchstick or finger (b).

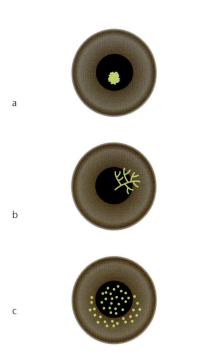

a

b

c

167 Corneal staining with fluorescein: abrasion (a) indicating superficial injury; dendrite (b) indicating herpes simplex; punctate staining (c) (many possible etiologies).

168 Determining the depth of the anterior chamber using the oblique flashlight test. A shadow cast on the nasal side of the iris indicates a shallow anterior chamber.

best to use sterile fluorescein on paper strips.) The epithelial defect will collect fluorescein dye and can be seen with the flashlight as greenish-yellow pooling. With blue light at the slit lamp, the dye in the defect will be bright green.

Fluorescein will identify these conditions, among others (**167**):

- Corneal abrasion.
- Herpes simplex (dendritic) keratitis (see also Figures 135, 136).
- Punctate spots on the cornea from trachoma, viral infections, corneal exposure, onchocerciasis, or leprosy.

Internal ocular examination

Two instruments are necessary to perform a good examination of the internal eye: a bright flashlight and a hand-held ophthalmoscope.

Check the depth of the anterior chamber by holding the flashlight on the lateral (temporal) side of the eye, parallel to the iris, and aimed across the eye (**168**). If the anterior chamber is of normal depth, there will be no shadow (darkening) on the nasal iris. If it is shallow, a shadow will be cast on the nasal iris. Note that pupillary dilation with cycloplegic eye drops in an eye with a shallow anterior chamber may cause acute ocular hypertension (see Angle closure glaucoma, Chapter 6).

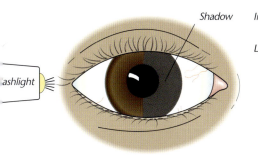

Shadow

Flashlight

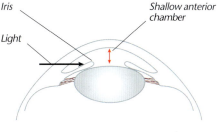

Iris

Light

Shallow anterior chamber

Check the pupillary reaction with the flashlight. The pupils should be equal in size and should constrict equally when the flashlight is directed into each pupil. If the pupil does not constrict when light is shone into the eye, the eye is probably not normal. Glaucoma is a common eye disease that causes the pupil to react poorly to light.

Examine the lens when checking the pupil. The lens may appear white or milky, evidence of a dense or mature cataract (see Chapter 5).

Opacities of the media and posterior segment disease can be identified using the ophthalmoscope. This last part of the examination should be performed in a dark room. The pupils should be dilated with tropicamide 1% or cyclopentolate 1%. Do not use atropine drops for pupillary dilation in routine examinations. A pupil dilated with atropine may remain dilated for up to 2 weeks, causing blurred vision.

Instruct the patient to stare straight ahead into the distance. Direct ophthalmoscopy is performed with the eye that corresponds to the eye being examined. Use the thumb of your free hand to raise the patient's upper eyelid.

Dial a +5 diopter lens into place in the aperture of the ophthalmoscope. Position the instrument approximately 20 cm (8 in) from the cornea until the red reflex (light reflected from the blood vessels of the choroid) comes into view.

Any opacity of the media will appear as a spot or interruption in the red reflex. If a dense opacity of the media is present (typically a mature cataract), then little or no red reflex will be seen. A faint corneal opacity, not visible during the external ocular examination, may be evident as an opacity of the media with this technique. Vitreous opacity should be suspected if a dull red reflex is present and there is neither a cataract nor a corneal opacity.

After examining for media opacities, move slowly closer to the patient's eye with the ophthalmoscope while dialing in smaller plus (+) lens numbers until the instrument is a few centimeters from the eyelids. Adjust the distance of the ophthalmoscope slightly back and forth until details of the retina come into focus.

Examine the optic nerve head (optic disc) first, noting its configuration and depth. Then examine the small arteries and veins that enter the retina from within the optic disc. Follow the vessels as far as possible with the ophthalmoscope light, looking for any abnormality.

Finally, examine the macula. To locate the macula, ask the patient to look directly at the light in the ophthalmoscope. A patient with good macular vision will look directly at the light with the macula. The macula will then be in full view.

Tonometry

Ocular tonometry is the measurement of intraocular pressure (IOP). Normal IOP is considered to be between 10–21 mm Hg. Elevated IOP can mean that the patient has glaucoma or is at risk of developing the condition (see Chapter 6). Accurate tonometry will help in diagnosing glaucoma. Tonometry should be performed on these patients.

- All patients over 40 years of age (all patients in sub-Saharan Africa and all people of African descent over 30 years of age because of the apparent earlier onset of open-angle glaucoma).
- Preoperative intraocular surgery patients.
- Postoperative intraocular surgery patients.
- Any patient in whom glaucoma is suspected.
- Any patient with unexplained visual loss.

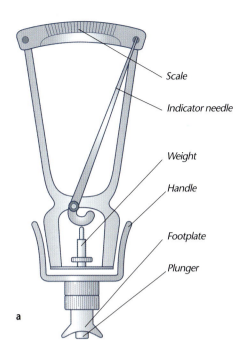

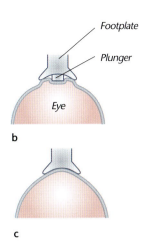

169 Tonometer indentation principle: diagram of the Schiøtz tonometer (a); tonometer plunger indents cornea – IOP is normal (<21 mmHg) (b); tonometer plunger indents cornea little or not at all – IOP is elevated (>21 mmHg) (c).

Schiøtz tonometry

The Schiøtz tonometer is a hand-held indentation tonometer that is convenient to use and widely available in the developing world. The principle of the indentation tonometer is simple: if the eye is hard (IOP elevated), the plunger in the tonometer indents the eye very little; if the IOP is normal or low, the plunger of the tonometer indents the eye more deeply (**169**). The amount of indentation of the eye is indicated by a number on the tonometer scale. This number is not the IOP. The IOP (in mmHg) is determined by converting the scale reading on the tonometer using a standard chart (included in the tonometer case and also see *Table 10*). The steps for performing Schiøtz tonometry are given overleaf.

Table 10 **Schiøtz tonometer scale**			
Tonometer reading (scale units)	Pressure (mmHg) according to load		
	5.5 g	7.5 g	20 g
0	41	59	81
1	35	50	69
2	29	42	59
3	24	36	51
4	21	30	43
5	17	26	37
6	15	22	32
7	12	19	27
8	10	16	23
9	9	13	20
10	7	11	17
11	6	9	14
12	5	8	12
13	4	6	10
14		5	8
15		4	6

Performing Schiøtz tonometry

1   Clean the tonometer footplate with cotton wool dipped in surgical spirits (e.g., methylated spirits) and dry it completely prior to use with every patient.

2   Position the patient on his or her back.

3   Place one drop of a topical anesthetic in the inferior fornix of each eye.

4   Instruct the patient to fixate in primary position on an overhead target. A convenient fixation target is the patient's thumb held above the face at arm's length. To record an accurate IOP the eyes must be still and must not move.

5   Retract the eyelids of the patient's right eye with the fingers of your left hand. (Opposite hands may be used according to the examiner's preference.) Your fingers should rest on the superior and inferior orbital rims and not on the eyelids. (Inaccurately high IOP readings will be obtained if the patient is squeezing the eyelids or if pressure from the examiner's fingers is transmitted to the eyeball through the eyelids.)

6   Hold the tonometer, fixed with the 5.5 g weight, in the right hand and bring it to the patient's right eye from the temporal side so as not to frighten or alarm the patient. Place the footplate gently on the center of the cornea. The pointer will move from its resting place. Note the scale reading of the tonometer and then remove the tonometer from the eye.

7   If the scale reading is 2 or less, replace the weight with the 7.5 g weight and repeat the measurement. If the reading is still less than 2, replace the weight with the 20 g weight and repeat the measurement.

8   Repeat the procedure on the left eye.

9   Convert the scale readings for the right and left eyes to IOP using the conversion chart.

10 Disassemble the tonometer and clean the footplate plunger and barrel at the end of each day's use of the instrument.

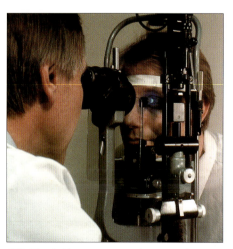

170 The Goldman tonometer is mounted on a slit lamp.

Applanation tonometry

This instrument measures IOP by flattening a constant area of the cornea. The weight required to do so is the IOP, measured in mmHg. The applanation tonometer is more accurate than the Schiøtz tonometer. It is usually mounted on a slit lamp (**170**), although a hand-held applanation tonometer is also available.

Tonopen

The tonopen is a hand-held tonometer. It is not as accurate as the slit lamp mounted applanation tonometer. Tonometry with a tonopen is quick and efficient when performed by a skilled eye health care worker (**171**).

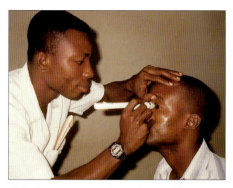

171 The tonopen can be used for rapid screening.

Examination of children

The examiner should be gentle and try to gain the child's confidence. An older child may be examined easily if the child is not afraid of the examiner.

Infants and uncooperative children may require physical restraint in order to perform an adequate ocular examination. There are several methods of restraining a child for examination (method 1 is better for older children; with infants, use method 2 or 3):

1. The examiner and an assistant sit opposite each other, close together. With the child's feet pointing toward the assistant, the assistant restrains the child's arms with one hand and legs with the other. The examiner immobilizes the child's head gently between his or her knees, leaving hands free to perform the examination.

2. Using the same position as above, the assistant draws the child's arms over the head with one hand so that the arms provide restraint at the sides of the head. With the other hand, the assistant restrains the legs (**172**).

3. The child can be wrapped (swaddled) securely in a blanket so that he or she is unable to move arms and legs (**173**).

If the child is squeezing his or her eyelids, retraction of the eyelids will be necessary to perform the examination. Eyelid retraction can be done with a retractor made from a paper clip (see Chapter 3).

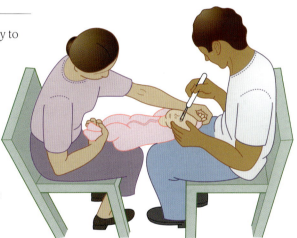

172 Restraining a child for ocular examination.

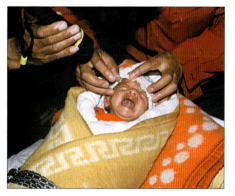

173 Restraining an infant with a blanket to facilitate examination.

Part 4

Appendices

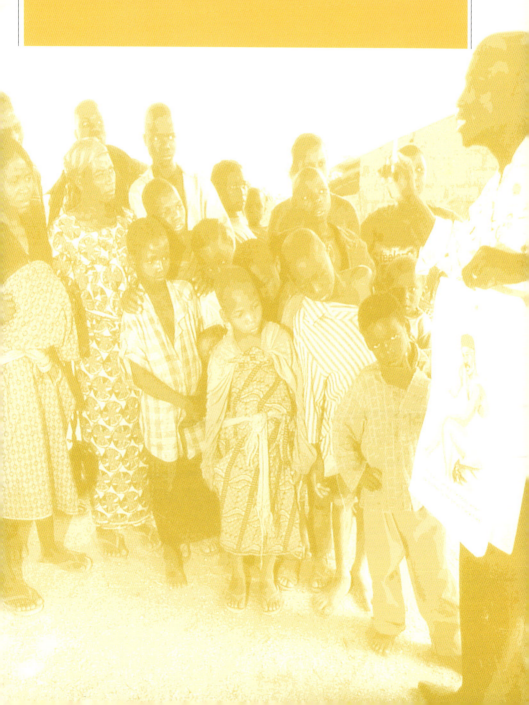

Appendix A

Diagnosis of the red eye

	Bacterial conjunctivitis	**Viral conjunctivitis**	**Allergic conjunctivitis**	**Active trachoma**
Occurrence	Common	Common	Common	May be very common in regions where trachoma is endemic
Discharge	Purulent	Watery with mucus	Usually minimal; may be watery	Purulent if bacterial infection is present
Symptoms	Discomfort; vision is decreased if cornea is involved	Discomfort; vision is decreased if cornea is involved	Itching without pain	Discomfort in early infection; pain if trichiasis also is present; decreased vision if corneal complications are present
IOP	Not affected	Not affected	Not affected	Not affected
Pupil	Normal	Normal	Normal	Normal
Conjunctiva	Red, often with papillary reaction	Diffusely red, with follicles	Papillary reaction	Papillary reaction and follicles
Involvement	One or both eyes	Usually both eyes	Usually both eyes	Usually both eyes
Lymph nodes	No adenopathy	Preauricular adenopathy	No adenopathy	No adenopathy
Staining with fluorescein	Usually no staining	Sometimes punctate staining	Usually no staining	Corneal staining if corneal complications are present

Herpes simplex (dendritic) keratitis	Acute iritis	Ocular surface trauma (cornea, conjunctiva, and sclera)	Acute (angle-closure) glaucoma	
Common	Common	Common	Uncommon; rare in Africa	**Occurrence**
None	None	Watery	None	**Discharge**
Pain and decreased vision	Pain and decreased vision	Pain and decreased vision	Pain and decreased vision	**Symptoms**
Not affected	Normal or low	Usually not affected	Elevated	**IOP**
Normal	Small and fixed to light	Normal	Dilated and fixed to light	**Pupil**
May be follicles and ciliary flush at limbus	Ciliary flush of limbal conjunctiva and sclera	Diffusely red	Diffusely red; cornea hazy	**Conjunctiva**
Usually one eye only	Usually one eye only	Usually one eye only; can be both with chemical injuries	Usually one eye only	**Involvement**
No adenopathy	No adenopathy	No adenopathy	No adenopathy	**Lymph nodes**
Typical dendritic branching	No corneal staining	Corneal staining with corneal or conjunctival abrasion	No corneal staining	**Staining with fluorescein**

Ocular medications

Essential ophthalmic drugs

The following is a suggested minimal list of medications for the practice of basic ophthalmology:

■ Tetracycline 1% ointment.
■ Chloramphenicol drops.
■ Atropine 1% drops or ointment.
■ Tropicamide 1% drops.
■ Hydrocortisone 0.5% drops or ointment.
■ Topical anesthetic.
■ Idoxuridine drops.
■ Pilocarpine 4% drops.
■ Acetazolamide 500-mg tablets.
■ Injectable corticosteroid (hydrocortisone).
■ Injectable anesthetic with adrenaline 1:10,000.
■ Fluorescein dye on filter paper strips.

Guidelines for usage of ophthalmic medications

■ Continue to use an ophthalmic drug only as long as necessary to achieve improvement or cure.
■ Teach the patient how to use prescribed ocular medications or teach a friend or relative of the patient how to administer medications to the patient
■ Topical medications should not be applied when a corneal or scleral perforation is known or suspected.
■ Never give topical anesthetics to patients for outpatient use.

■ Corticosteroids should only be prescribed with great caution. Use these medications only when correctly indicated and do not prescribe them for red or painful eyes without knowing the diagnosis.
■ Corticosteroids should not be given to patients for 'itchy' or 'burning' eyes. If the diagnosis is uncertain, it is better to use a decongestant, such as zinc sulfate.
■ Atropine should not be used to dilate the pupil for funduscopy because of its long-lasting effects. Use shorter-acting medications, such as tropicamide 1%, phenylephrine 10%, or cyclopentolate 1%.
■ By international standards, bottles with red caps contain drops that dilate the pupil (mydriatics and cycloplegics, such as cyclopentolate, tropicamide, phenylephrine, homatropine, and atropine). Bottles with green caps contain drugs that constrict the pupil (miotics, such as pilocarpine and physostigmine).
■ To conserve medications, apply only the minimal amount needed to the eye. The correct way to apply drops is to retract the lower eyelid slightly with a clean finger and apply one drop only to the inferior fornix. Be careful not to touch the eyelid or eyeball with the tip of the bottle. Likewise, only a small amount of ointment is necessary, applied in the same way.

Guidelines for use of corticosteroids

Topical corticosteroids have at least five effects on the human eye. Four of these effects are potentially blinding; the fifth is a beneficial effect. Corticosteroids can do the following:

- Cause herpes simplex virus to become active and invade the cornea.
- Create an ideal setting for fungal keratitis, especially when applied to the eye following a corneal foreign body of vegetable matter.
- Cause posterior subcapsular cataract.
- Produce secondary open-angle glaucoma.
- Reduce ocular inflammation when used according to proper indications.

Corticosteroids used to treat eye diseases can be dangerous. To avoid blinding complications in the use of topical corticosteroids, good clinical judgment must be used. Note the following points:

- Do not use a corticosteroid drop or ointment on a corneal abrasion.
- Do not use a corticosteroid drop or ointment to treat a 'red eye' when the diagnosis is not known.
- Never use a corticosteroid drop or ointment on a herpes simplex dendritic ulcer.
- Do not use a corticosteroid drop or ointment on a confirmed bacterial corneal ulcer.
- Do not use a corticosteroid drop or ointment on 'allergic conjunctivitis' if a true allergic situation is not present.

Corticosteroids are appropriate for use in the following situations:

- Tarsal and limbal vernal conjunctivitis.
- Keratitis of a non-herpetic and non-infectious nature.
- Uveitis (including iritis, iridocyclitis, cyclitis, and choroiditis).
- Extraocular and intraocular postoperative inflammation. If the diagnosis has not been established, it is better to use an antibiotic drop that does not contain a corticosteroid preparation. If corticosteroids are indicated and are being used properly, the eye should be checked regularly for posterior subcapsular cataract, dendritic (herpetic) keratitis, fungal keratitis, corneal ulcer, and secondary ocular hypertension.

The blind, painful eye

For blind and painful eyes that do not respond to analgesics, enucleation may be performed to eliminate pain. If the patient does not agree to enucleation, retrobulbar alcohol may be administered for permanent pain relief as follows:

1 Inject 1.0 cc of local anesthetic (e.g., lidocaine) into the retrobulbar space.
2 Leave the retrobulbar needle in place and remove the syringe.
3 Draw up 2.0 cc of 100% alcohol (ethanol) into the syringe with a separate needle.
4 Inject the absolute alcohol through the retrobulbar needle into the retrobulbar space.
5 Leave the retrobulbar needle in place and remove the syringe.
6 Draw up 1.0 cc of local anesthetic into the syringe with a separate needle.
7 Inject the local anesthetic into the retrobulbar space as the needle is slowly withdrawn.

■ If a prescribed drug is not achieving its desired effect, or if the eye becomes worse while undergoing treatment, you can suspect that the patient may also be applying non-prescribed medication. In particular, many drugs, herbs, and remedies supplied by traditional healers may be used by patients at the same time that they are undergoing treatment by eye health care workers. Many of those preparations may produce irritation and redness of the conjunctiva. Some preparations may be toxic and can cause corneal damage and permanent blindness. In taking a history from a patient who has a red or irritated eye, ask about the use of traditional medications. These may be prescribed by a traditional healer or they may be prepared by the patient or the family.

Appendix C

Surgical guidelines for ophthalmic medical auxiliaries

Surgical indications

- A corneal laceration should be repaired immediately upon diagnosis.
- Lacerations involving the face and eyelids should be repaired immediately upon diagnosis.
- Any mature or hypermature cataract in a monocular or binocular cataract patient should be extracted because of the risk of phacotoxic uveitis and glaucoma.
- Bilateral mature or hypermature cataracts should be extracted as soon as possible.

Preoperative: cataract patients

- If the cataract is not mature, dilate the pupil and do a fundus examination. Carefully examine the macula, the retina, and the optic disc.
- If you cannot see through a cataract to examine the fundus, the patient's vision is significantly impaired. Cataract extraction is indicated.
- Perform tonometry on all preoperative patients.
- If you are in doubt about whether surgery is indicated, consult an ophthalmologist.
- All surgery on one-eyed patients should be performed only by an ophthalmologist.

Preoperative: open-angle glaucoma patients

- Perform screening tonometry.
- After tonometry has been performed, dilate the pupil for fundus examination of the optic disc.
- If primary open-angle glaucoma is present, administer 4% pilocarpine every 6 hr until surgery can be performed.
- If the glaucoma is secondary, treat the primary cause. If the cause is iritis, avoid the use of miotics; treat with acetazolamide, corticosteroids, and atropine 1%.

Preoperative: cataract and glaucoma

- Perform an eye examination, including tonometry and examination of the ocular fundus.
- Wash the patient's face daily. If the patient is hospitalized, face washing should be a daily routine while awaiting surgery.
- Apply atropine 1% daily to the eye awaiting surgery.
- Apply tetracycline 1% eye ointment daily to the eye awaiting surgery.
- Obtain an operative permit from the patient and/or the patient's family.

Basic equipment

Basic instruments and supplies

A basic surgical instrumentation and sterilizing kit and a list of expendable supplies for performing intraocular surgery – including ICCE, ECCE/IOL, and glaucoma surgery – is listed below. This equipment should be packed in sturdy containers and can be used in mobile eye surgery and rural hospital work:

- 10-cc syringe
- 2-cc syringe
- 21-gauge needles
- 27-gauge needles
- Peribulbar needles
- Cannula for irrigation of fornices
- Small smooth wire eyelid retractor
- Locking needle holder for 4-0 bridle suture
- Muscle hook
- Forceps (for grasping superior rectus for bridle suture)
- Mosquito forceps
- Fine-pointed scissors
- Blunt-tipped scissors (optional)
- Blade breaker and holder and carbon-steel razor blades
- Surgical blade handle and blades
- Bishop–Harmon (or similar toothed) tissue forceps
- Alcohol flame lamp and ball-tipped thermal cautery, or battery-powered cautery

- Right- and left-handed corneoscleral scissors, or universal corneoscleral scissors
- Graefe knife (optional)
- Fine-needle holder for 8-0 to 10-0 suture
- Fine suturing forceps (Colibri or other)
- Iris forceps (optional: Colibri forceps can be used)
- Iris scissors (Dewecker or other)
- Smooth nontoothed forceps
- IOL forceps (for implantation)
- Lens-dialing instrument (Sinsky hook)
- Capsule scissors (Vannas)
- Two-way manual aspiration/irrigation set (Simcoe or McIntyre)
- Iris retractor and expressor
- Scleral punch
- One or more cataract extraction tools:
    - Erysiphake with spare bulbs
    - Capsule forceps
    - Silica gel pellets
    - Portable cryoextractor
    - Lens loop
    - Cystotome (may be made by bending tip of 30-gauge needle with mosquito forceps)
- Air injection cannula
- Portable sterilizing unit (for example, gas stove)
- Stainless steel basins for boiling
- Shallow stainless steel basin for sterilizing sharp instruments in chemical solution
- Methyl alcohol and/or acetone
- Small stainless steel cup for sterile solution on surgical tray

Sterile gowns, drapes, and towels

Stainless steel drums for storing and transporting sterile gowns, drapes, and towels

Three towel clips

Portable headrest

Sterile cellulose sponges

Registration book for surgical operations

Surgical loupes: 2.5 power to 4.0 power (depending on surgeon's preference)

Selection of posterior chamber and anterior chamber IOLs

Viscoelastic (sterile methylcellulose in syringes)

4-0 bridle suture

9-0, 10-0 suture

Alpha-chymotrypsin

Millipore filters

Acetazolamide 500-mg tablets

Chloramphenicol 1% drops (readily available in many developing countries)

Tropicamide 1%

Proparacaine topical anesthetic drops

Lidocaine hydrochloride 1% or 2%

Timolol maleate 0.5%

(See also Appendix B for essential ocular medications.)

Care of instruments and equipment

All sharp and delicate intraocular instruments must be protected from damage. They must be handled gently at all times. Storage on a flat tray with each instrument secured by elastic binding is advisable.

Sterilization of instruments can be achieved by boiling or with a steam autoclave. Sharp instruments and scissors should be lightly but thoroughly cleaned after every surgical session with a soft brush and surgical spirits (methyl alcohol or acetone) rather than boiled. Proper cleaning and storage prolong the life of surgical instruments.

The tonometer, the ophthalmoscope, the slit lamp, and the operating microscope should be covered when not in use to protect them from dust and debris. Hand instruments should be stored in their cases until they are next used; cloth or plastic covers should be used for slit lamps and portable operating microscopes if portable cases are not available.

Spare bulbs and fuses for battery-powered and electrically powered instruments should be available. No battery-powered instrument should be stored for a long period of time containing its batteries. Old and leaking batteries will damage instruments.

In wet climates, examination instruments – particularly ophthalmoscopes – should be regularly inspected for mildew. These instruments should be cleaned regularly with a soft, dry cotton cloth.

Schiøtz tonometers should be stored clean and dry. A wire and cotton cleaner (a pipe cleaner used for cleaning tobacco pipes) soaked in surgical spirits or acetone is excellent for cleaning the barrel of the tonometer. Allow the barrel to air dry and then wipe it with a soft cotton cloth. The Schiøtz tonometer should be disassembled for storage in its case and reassembled before using; this prevents the shaft from sticking to the barrel.

Equipment suppliers

This is a partial list of companies that sell ophthalmic surgical instruments and equipment at prices known to be less than those of more well-known international companies. The equipment, although less expensive, is durable and good to excellent in quality. Contact details correct at time of going to press.

Surgical instruments

Dixey Instruments Limited

5 High Street
Brixworth
Northants
NN6 9DD
UK
Tel: +44-1604 882480
Fax: +44-1604 882488

Dixey Instruments manufactures and supplies a wide range of high-quality surgical instruments and equipment.

Indo-German Surgical Corporation

123 Kaliandas Udyue Bhavan
Near Century Bazar
Prabhadevi
Post Box No. 19129
Mumbai 400 025
India

Indian manufacturer of ophthalmic surgical instruments and appliances. Recommended by experienced ophthalmic consultants.

Suzhou Medical Instrument Company

34 Daru Lane
Suzhou
Jiangsu 215005
China
Fax: +86-512-5244789

A company that manufactures surgical instruments, operating microscopes, and other ophthalmic equipment.

Operating microscopes

Microsurgery should be performed through co-axial illumination microscopes with variable magnification. Microscopes are available through the Indo-German Surgical Corporation and the Suzhou Medical Instrument Company.

Scan Optics

30/32 Sterling Street
Thebarton SA5031
Australia
Tel: +61-6188-234 9120
Fax: +61-6188-234 9417

Scan Optics manufactures and distributes a high-quality and reasonably priced portable and compact operating micro-scope especially designed and built for outreach and rural work.

Leica

Ernst-Leitz-Strasse 17?37
Leica Microsystems AG
35578 Wetzlar
Germany
Fax: +49-64-41292590
www.MicroscopeStore.com

Leica operating systems are of very high quality and considerably more expensive than Scan Optics, Indo-German, and Suzhou Medical Instrument Company instruments.

Carl Zeiss

Surgical Product Division
73446 Oberkochen
Germany
Fax: +49-73-64204823
E-mail: surgical@zeiss.de
www.zeiss.com/eye

Zeiss operating microscopes are of high quality and considerably more expensive than Scan Optics, Indo-German, and Suzhou Medical Instrument Company instruments.

Magnifying operating loupes (spectacles)

Available through the Indo-German Surgical Corporation and the Suzhou Optical Company and:

Keeler

Clewer Hill Road
Windsor
Berkshire SL4 4AA
UK

Heine

Kientalstrasse
78036 Herrsching
Germany

Operating theater lights

Daray Lighting Limited

7 Commerce Way
Stanbridge Road
Leighton Buzzard
Bedforshire LU7 8RW
UK
Tel: +44-1525 376766
Fax: +44-1525 851626

Daray manufactures a portable, durable operating light that is powered by both a 12-volt vehicle battery or mains electrical supply.

Portable Cryoprobes

Restored Sight Projects, Ltd

Singleton Court
Monastow Road
Monmouth NP5 3AH
UK
Tel: 44-1600 716911

This company manufactures a small portable cryoprobe.

Bright Instrument Company Ltd
St. Margarets Way
Stukeley Meadows
Huntingdon
Cambridgeshire PE18 6ED
UK
Tel: 44-1480 454528

Bright Instrument Company manufactures small gas substitute cylinders that are ozone friendly for use with handheld cryoprobes.

Autoclaves

LTE Scientific Ltd
Greenbridge Lane
Greenfield
Oldham OL3 7EN
UK
Tel: +44-1457 876221
Fax: +44-1457 870131

LTE Scientific manufactures a range of high-quality surgical autoclaves.

Hyaluronidase
This enzyme is available in powdered form and improves the distribution of injected local anesthesia. It has become difficult to obtain but may be ordered from:

CP Pharmaceuticals Ltd
Ash Road
North Wrexham Industrial Estate
Wrexham LL13 9UF
UK
Tel: +44-1978 6611261
Fax: +44-1978 660130

Rallis India
Pharmaceutical Division
B-9/2 M.I.D.C.
Waluj 431136
India

Appendix F

WHO classification of visual impairment and blindness

Category of visual impairment	Visual acuity with best possible correction	
	Maximum less than:	Minimum equal to or better than:
1	6/18 m 20/60 ft	6/60 m 20/200 ft
2	6/60 20/200	3/60 (finger counting at 3 m) 20/400
3	3/60 (finger counting at 3 m) 20/400	1/60 (finger counting at 1 m) 20/1200
4	1/60 (finger counting at 1m) 20/1200	Light perception
5	No light perception	No light perception

Low vision — categories 1 and 2

Blindness — categories 3, 4 and 5

Resource organizations

The following are summaries of a range of international organizations involved in blindness prevention and sight restoration. For a more complete list and further contact details, see Appendix H.

Aravind Eye Care System

Mission

Upon his retirement from government service at the age of 58, Dr. V (Dr. G. Venkataswamy) founded the Aravind Eye Hospital in 1976. Its mission is to eliminate needless blindness by providing appropriate, compassionate, and high-quality eye care to all patients.

Ever since its inception, Dr. V's passionate commitment toward this mission has been Aravind's driving force. His relentless efforts have resulted in the establishment of Aravind Eye Care System (AECS), which comprises a network of five hospitals with a total capacity of 3600 beds, a comprehensive outreach network, an education and training facility (LAICO) exclusively to teach and train eye care workers, and a manufacturing facility (Aurolab) that provides high-quality ophthalmic supplies at costs affordable to developing economies. The service area of the five hospitals covers a population of about 90 million in the states of Tamil Nadu and Kerala in India.

Strong leadership and a value system composed of compassion, equity, and transparency govern the operation of the Aravind system. The key areas are those of patient access, productivity, quality, finance, and human resources. The central principle of the model is to proactively generate patient flow and achieve high productivity while ensuring that high-quality standards are met.

Activities and programs

Through the coordinated contribution of a committed staff, Aravind continues to be the largest provider of eye care services and trainer of eye care personnel in the world. Aravind Eye Hospitals handle over 1.6 million outpatient visits and perform close to 250,000 surgeries annually. Two-thirds of its services are offered free or at steeply subsidized rates and are funded primarily through the revenues from its paying patients.

Recognizing that many rural communities and poor people are unable to, or simply do not, access eye care for reasons such as lack of awareness, logistics, or finances, Aravind pioneered the concept of eye screening camps, held in partnership with local community groups. Patients receive comprehensive eye exams and those who require glasses get them on the spot at an affordable cost. Those requiring surgery are transported to the nearest Aravind Eye Hospital. There they receive free of cost the surgery, stay, food, and medication required after discharge, return transport, and follow-up after 6 weeks. Each year about 1300 such eye-screening camps are held, through which close to 100,000 surgeries are performed.

Higher volume brings down the cost and ensures both affordability and viability of the enterprise. Volume in turn is ensured by the combination of low cost, high quality, and efficient procedures, as well as the appropriate use of human resources and technology.

Aravind, through its division LAICO (Lions Aravind Institute of Community Ophthalmology), actively shares its knowledge and systems with other eye care providers to help them enhance their effectiveness. Over 200 eye hospitals from India and other developing countries have participated in this process.

Through Aurolab, another arm of the Aravind Eye Care System, eye care is made affordable by its production and supply of high-quality ophthalmic supplies at affordable cost to over 120 developing countries. Aravind Eye Care System is now offering management contracting services to run eye hospitals in underserved areas and a beginning has been made with managing two eye hospitals in eastern and northern India. Its work and continued efforts are revolutionizing hundreds of eye care programs in developing countries.

Aurolab

Making quality eye care affordable
Aravind Eye Care System has consistently challenged the boundaries of its primary scope of activities – quality eye care at affordable rates – to successfully venture into related areas such as the manufacture of eye care products. In response to a growing need for affordable use of IOLs in cataract surgery, and to fulfill the organizational goal of eradicating needless blindness, Aravind Eye Care System established Aurolab in 1991 as a charitable trust to initially develop and manufacture inexpensive intraocular lenses (IOLs). It later diversified into the manufacture of suture needles, pharmaceutical products, blades, and other instruments.

Aurolab manufactures a variety of three-piece, single-piece, and foldable lenses, the complete range of non-absorbable and absorbable ophthalmic sutures, and a wide range of surgical adjuncts, eye drops, and other pharmaceutical products. Aurolab also offers *The Cataract Kit*, a customized pack of all surgical supplies required for five cataract surgeries. Aurolab uses state-of-the-art technology in its production facilities and has an efficient distribution system enabling it to market IOLs, suture needles, and pharmaceutical products in India and 120 countries worldwide. It is targeted primarily at non-profit and government organizations.

Aravind Eye Care System has also initiated a hugely successful IOL surgery training program to help ophthalmologists make the transition from conventional surgery to microsurgery.

Aurolab's recognition as supplier of world-class quality products with a strong customer focus is evidenced by the ISO 9001:2000 certification for its quality systems and product certification by CE.

Aurolab continues to evolve to address the increasing need for other affordable ophthalmic supplies and equipment through innovations in its product lines, while working with distribution partners across the world to reach a broader spectrum of the underserved population.

The Carter Center (TCC)

Activities and programs

The Carter Center's international health programs, which are focused on visual health, include the River Blindness Program and Trachoma Program. Through the River Blindness Program, The Carter Center has assisted in the delivery of more than 70 million treatments of Mectizan® in Africa and Latin America as of January 2006. The Trachoma Control Program has seven programs in six African countries that work with Ministries of Health to fight blinding trachoma. The Carter Center is the lead organization focusing on the Facial cleanliness and Environmental improvement aspects of the WHO SAFE strategy for trachoma control.

Educational materials

Trachoma health education materials used in Carter Center programs are available via the TCC website(www.cartercenter.org).

Christoffel-Blindenmission/ Christian Blind Mission (CBM)

The Christoffel-Blindenmission (Christian Blind Mission) is an international Christian organization that supports programs for persons with disabilities in developing countries. Its aim is to improve the quality of life of persons with disabilities by:

- Providing medical health care services.
- Providing rehabilitation and education.
- Advocating the inclusion of people with disabilities as equals in all aspects of society.

In 2005 CBM supported 1019 projects in 113 countries in Africa, Asia, Latin America, and Eastern Europe with a total program budget of almost EUR 50 million.

Activities and programs

The prevention and cure of blindness being traditionally the most important field of work, CBM also supports the education and rehabilitation of people with physical, mental, or intellectual disabilities and programs for people with hearing loss.

The CBM supports programs for people with visual loss in the following areas:

- Prevention of blindness.
- Low vision care.
- Education of visually impaired people.

Campaigns and cooperations

The CBM cooperates with global institutions and contributes to international campaigns. The CBM has been recognized as a professional organization for people with disabilities by the World Health Organization (WHO) and obtained roster consultative status with the United Nations Economic and Social Council.

As a member of the International Agency of Prevention of Blindness (IAPB), and in cooperation with WHO, the CBM has launched Vision 2020: The Right to Sight. The goal of Vision 2020 is to eliminate avoidable blindness by the year 2020.

Working principles and structures

The CBM implements its programs through local partners which are supported with financial resources, expertise, and sufficient staff. Twelve regional offices assist partner organizations in the provision of services to people with disabilities. The CBM cooperates with a broad group of international disability experts who provide technical knowledge and consultancy services in all fields of work. The CBM member associations in ten countries raise funds and advocate for the support of the overseas programs.

Dana Center for Preventive Ophthalmology

Aims and provisions

The Dana Center, an integral division within the Department of Ophthalmology, Wilmer Institute, at the Johns Hopkins University School of Medicine, Baltimore, consists of faculty and staff devoted to a public health approach in prevention of visual impairment worldwide. Founded by Alfred Sommer and Hugh Taylor in 1981, it is a collaborating center for the World Health Organization, providing consultation and expertise in blindness and vision care programs in every part of the world.

Activities and programs

The Dana Center has ophthalmologists, epidemiologists, biostatisticians, and field project specialists. Its work includes programs that address the problems of cataract, glaucoma, trachoma, nutritional blindness, and pediatric eye disease. Its present programs include prevalence surveys, clinical trials, programs applying present care to developing countries, technology assessment, and disease modeling. Areas in which direct research or service studies have been conducted include Eastern Europe, Africa, the Middle East, India, Nepal, China, Mexico, and South America.

The Dana Center is available for interactive consultation and programs with individuals and other groups for subjects of common interest. Funding is obtained on a case-by-case basis from governmental, non-governmental charity, and private sources.

Education

Several educational programs are provided by the Dana Center. Every three years, the Public Health Ophthalmologist Program is conducted in collaboration with the Hopkins Bloomberg School of Public Health. Ophthalmologists/students who are typically not citizens of the USA matriculate in this course for one year, leading to the Master of Public Health degree, and return to their home country to continue work in public health ophthalmology. United States citizens are offered multi-year fellowship opportunities through the NIH-funded Clinician-Scientist programs (K awards). These mentored training programs include course work and practical development of research skills related to epidemiological and public health projects. Most people who enter this training are expected to remain within full-time faculty status. In addition to these major programs, individual fellowships of one or more years have been arranged for people who desire more experience in public health ophthalmology. Medical students and doctoral candidates are often accommodated within existing research programs in the USA or elsewhere as junior participants.

For more information, visit the website:
Public Health Ophthalmologist Program:
http://www.hopkinsmedicine.org/wilmer/education/dana.html
Clinician-Scientist Training Program:
http://www.hopkinsmedicine.org/wilmer/education/clinicial_scientist1.html

Fred Hollows Foundation

Activities and programs

The Fred Hollows Foundation (FHF) facilitates international eye health programs in Africa, Asia, Australia, and the Pacific. Developed and implemented through active collaborations with local organizations, these programs achieve the following:

- Provide training and development for various health professionals, including ophthalmologists, ophthalmic nurses, hospital administrators, and village volunteers.
- Screen for and treat blinding eye conditions of disadvantaged people from remote communities.
- Promote information sharing among local program partners and medical advisers in each country, within regions and throughout the FHF network.
- Advocate for change in the perception, policy, and priority of eye health issues.
- Support the upgrade of physical infrastructure and surgical equipment in local hospitals and community health facilities.
- Build the capacity of local partner organizations.

Volunteering

People interested in getting involved with the work of the FHF can do so through the following means:

- International Mentoring and Fund-Raising program (linking like-minded health professionals in a volunteer educational relationship).
- See the World Challenge (for intrepid travelers seeking a unique and life-changing experience).

- I Care day, The Miracle Club, and the Rotary Down Under Joint Partnership (for financial support with a difference).
- Special arrangements: contact the organization directly; it may be possible to volunteer or visit the programs.

Resources

Web-based resources include: individual profiles of people, programs, and partnerships; corporate (annual report, strategic framework) and technical publications; resources about Fred Hollows and The Foundation for school audiences; more information and opportunities to make a donation; and some very useful means to demonstrate support (e-cards, wallpapers, screensavers, buttons, etc.).

For more information see the website: www.hollows.org.

Foundation of the American Academy of Ophthalmology (FAAO)

The FAAO's International Assistance program contributes to the education of ophthalmologists in developing nations and facilitates international volunteerism.

Educational materials

Ophthalmic educational materials are provided free to ophthalmology residency programs in low-income nations. In addition, a manual is provided to each resident at selected institutions.

Educational opportunities

The Rotary Club Host Project, a partnership of FAAO and Rotary Clubs, brings selected ophthalmologists from developing nations to the USA for a 2-week educational experience that includes attending the AAO Annual Meeting.

International volunteerism

The EyeCare Volunteer Registry, www.eye-carevolunteer.org, is an Internet-based program that links eye care professionals interested in volunteering with organizations and institutions that need assistance. EyeCare Volunteers provide educational and clinical services in developing nations.

Resources

Publications available on the FAAO website (www.faao.org) include the following:

– *Before You Go: Information for Ophthalmologists Volunteering in Developing Nations*
– *Guidelines for Ophthalmologists Volunteering in Developing Nations*
– *Publications on Ophthalmology in Developing Nations*
– *Ocular Considerations in Disaster Relief*
– *Buyer's Guide: Purchasing Ophthalmic Equipment in Developing Nations*

Helen Keller International (HKI)

Mission

Helen Keller International's mission is to save the sight and lives of the most vulnerable and disadvantaged people. They combat the causes and consequences of blindness and malnutrition by establishing programs based on evidence and research in vision, health, and nutrition. They strive to be a most scientifically competent non-profit organization in improving health and nutrition throughout the world.

Activities and programs

The Helen Keller International Program operates in three regions (Africa, Asia, and the Americas), encompassing 25 nations and directly benefiting millions of people each year. The two major areas of focus are (a) eye health and (b) health and nutrition.

Cataract

Helen Keller International promotes timely detection of eye problems, with an emphasis on childhood and adult cataract, in order to provide efficient delivery of intervention. They train surgeons, nurses, and community health workers, and develop basic eye health education programs with government counterparts and local non-governmental organizations, also providing the equipment and technology necessary for program implementation.

Onchocerciasis

HKI distributes an annual dose of Mectizan®, courtesy of Merck & Co., Inc, and works to provide communities across Africa with information and education about the prevention and treatment of the disease.

Trachoma

HKI works to end this disease of poverty with community-based approaches such as enhanced school health and female literacy training. These programs are linked through partnerships for environmental improvements such as school water supply and latrine construction. Surgical training and provision of needed antibiotic supplies and equipment strengthen and empower struggling government health service systems.

ChildSight®
Bringing Education into FocusTM

ChildSight® is HKI's domestic initiative which serves children living in urban and rural poverty and addresses refractive error, a visual problem that occurs in 25% of children aged 10–15. Prescription eyeglasses are the simple, immediate solution to this common problem. ChildSight® offers free vision screenings and free eyeglasses to children who need them. The connection between vision and academic improvement is dramatic and life-changing. Due to the success of the program, it is now active in Indonesia, Mexico, Morocco, and South Africa, with plans for further expansion.

Nutrition

Vitamin-A supplementation is one of the most cost-effective methods of preventing blindness in children, costing about one dollar per person each year. HKI focuses on vitamin-A supplementation, nutrition education, promoting the consumption of vitamin-A-rich foods, homestead food production, and encouraging food fortification with micronutrients.

IAPB and VISION 2020

Vision

A world in which no one is needlessly blind and where those with unavoidable vision loss can achieve their full potential.

Mission

To eliminate the main causes of avoidable blindness by the year 2020 by facilitating the planning, development and implementation of sustainable national eye care programs based on the three core strategies of disease control, human resource development and infrastructure development incorporating the principles of primary health care.

This will be achieved by mobilizing the will and passion for action through advocacy and through the mobilization of resources.

Introduction

In the mid-1970s, the late Sir John Wilson, amongst others, began to draw the international community's attention to the problem of global blindness. These efforts led to the setting up of the International Agency for the Prevention of Blindness (IAPB) on 1 January 1975, with Sir John Wilson as the Founder President. IAPB was established as a coordinating, umbrella organization to lead an international effort to promote blindness prevention activities. IAPB aspired to link the following groups with national programs for the prevention of blindness:

- Professional bodies
- Non-Governmental Organisations (NGOs)
- Educational institutions
- Interested individuals.

The first major achievement of IAPB was to promote the establishment of a WHO Programme for Prevention of Blindness (WHO/PBL), with which it then entered into official relationships.

Between 1996 and 1998, through a series of consultations between the Programme Advisory Group (PAG) of WHO, the Partnership Committee (an informal group of NGOs) and the IAPB Task Force, the document *Global Initiative for the Elimination of Avoidable Blindness* was developed and adopted. This set out priorities and strategies to eliminate avoidable blindness by the year 2020.

The joint program VISION 2020: The Right to Sight was officially launched by WHO, in Geneva in February 1999, and further promoted by IAPB at the sixth Assembly in Beijing in September 1999.

Rationale

In the 1990s, available data showed that:
- At least 75% of blindness was among the poor and very poor.
- At least 75% of blindness was the result of five conditions, each of which had a cost-effective means of prevention or cure.

- The number of people blind or at risk of blindness was far greater than could be managed by available services for the prevention and treatment of blindness.
- The shortfall in the supply of such services against the demand for them was widening at an ever-increasing rate.
- The humanitarian and economic costs of this situation were unacceptably high.

VISION 2020 therefore was conceived as a global movement to push governments to recognise the costs of avoidable blindness and to allocate resources to ensure that all people had access to good eye care services.

Activities and programs

The launch of VISION 2020 has led to concerted international effort in advocacy, resource mobilisation, joint planning, strengthening national capacities through human resource development and the transfer of appropriate technologies to developing countries. IAPB's main activities are listed below.

- Developing global technical plans highlighting the priority areas that need to be addressed in each region and the proposed strategies to reach the goals of VISION 2020 in these regions.
- Resource mobilization activities to increase the availability of funds to support prevention of blindness programs.
- Organizing regional and national VISION 2020 workshops and launch events in WHO/IAPB regions to raise awareness of blindness prevention and develop national and district level plans for prevention of blindness.

- Advocacy, primarily through global World Sight Day celebrations, initiated by the SightFirst Campaign of Lions Club International Foundation, and held on the second Thursday of October every year.
- Regional programs to control onchocerciasis and trachoma. These bring together critical components like accurate data, cost-effective interventions and partnerships.
- IAPB working groups such as the Human Resource Working Group and Low Vision Working Group aim to address lacunae in their relevant areas of interest. Training programs supported by IAPB help build critical mass in human resources, tailored to meet regional requirements.
- Training programs; for example, on pediatric ophthalmology and eye care management.
- Encouragement of private sector participation. For example, Carl Zeiss Training Centers are to be established to develop centers of excellence and support from Standard Chartered Bank will provide one million sight restorations over three years.

In May 2003, the 56th World Health Assembly of Ministers adopted a Resolution on Elimination of Avoidable Blindness, which calls on all member states to prepare VISION 2020 plans by 2005. In response to the Resolution, a VISION 2020 Tool Kit has been developed to provide guidance and support for governments and health professionals.

The new structure and constitution adopted by IAPB in September 2004 will help accelerate efforts to eliminate avoidable blindness, capitalizing on the momentum already created by the VISION 2020: The Right to Sight initiative, through the combined efforts of all the partners in this endeavor.

International Centre for Eye Health (ICEH)

Mission

The International Centre for Eye Health, now based at the London School of Hygiene and Tropical Medicine, was established to address the need of developing countries for expertise in blindness prevention.

The ICEH, a World Health Organization Collaborating Centre for Prevention of Blindness, aims to empower eye health workers to deliver high-quality eye care to people living in the poorest and most remote rural communities in the world, in order to eliminate avoidable blindness.

Activities and programs

The ICEH is unique worldwide in its three key activities:

- *Research* into the main blinding diseases and their treatment.
- *Training* of eye health workers from low-income countries.
- *Information and education* for eye health workers worldwide.

Research

The ICEH's research program focuses on the VISION 2020 priorities. It has identified the specific barriers to uptake of eye care services and, through long-term partnership with local eye care providers and community groups, aims to change people's attitudes toward blindness as well as restore sight.

Training

Courses in Community Eye Health are offered at Masters and Diploma level. Shorter courses – Control of Blinding Diseases, Planning a VISION 2020 Programme, and Tropical Ophthalmology – are also available.

The VISION 2020 Links Programme is designed to give institutions in developing countries the skills and resources to develop high-quality training and services through a link with a UK institution.

Information and education

The *Community Eye Health Journal* is produced quarterly and distributed free to developing countries. It is available in English (with an Indian supplement within India), French, and Chinese, and has a circulation of around 15,000 to approximately 75 countries.

The ICEH Resource Centre produces teaching materials in various formats, some of which are downloadable from the website, and provides distribution and information services. It has been instrumental in the development of Regional Resource Centres in South Africa, Tanzania, Nigeria, Colombia, India, and Pakistan.

For more information visit the following websites:
www.iceh.org.uk
www.jceh.co.uk

International Council of Ophthalmology (ICO)/ International Federation of Ophthalmological Societies (IFOS)

Introduction
The International Federation of Ophthalmological Societies (IFOS) represents and serves professional associations of ophthalmologists throughout the world. The ICO is its executive body and operational arm.

The roots of IFOS and the ICO date back to 1857 when 150 ophthalmologists from 24 countries convened in Brussels for the first International Congress of Ophthalmology. Participants in the Congress founded the ICO in 1927 in Scheveningen, Holland, and IFOS in 1933 in Madrid, Spain.

Mission
The ICO works with ophthalmologic societies, ophthalmologists and others to enhance ophthalmic education and the provision of eye care in order to preserve and protect vision for all people worldwide.

Aims
- Enhancing ophthalmic education, particularly training of ophthalmologists and other eye care personnel to meet public needs in developing countries.
- Stimulating and supporting communication and collaboration among ophthalmologic societies and ophthalmologists globally and their involvement in initiatives to preserve vision.
- Defining and disseminating proposed standards and guidelines in order to enhance eye care.
- Stimulating research to eradicate preventable blindness.
- Raising awareness worldwide of the economic, social and personal impact of vision loss and advocating for increased funding and other support for preservation and restoration of vision.

Activities and programs
The principle programs and activities of the ICO include the following:

- The International Congress of Ophthalmology, also called the World Ophthalmology Congress, which is held every two years in a different region of the world.
- The ICO International Basic Science Assessment and Clinical Sciences Assessment for Ophthalmologists.
- IFOS/ICO International Fellowship.
- ICO International Clinical Guidelines.
- Other ICO initiatives in ophthalmic education.
- Advocacy for preservation of vision.
- Vision for the Future, the International Ophthalmology Strategic Plan to Preserve and Restore Vision.
- Research Agenda for Global Blindness Prevention.
- The Eye Site and other communications initiatives.

International Eye Foundation (IEF)

Mission

The International Eye Foundation is dedicated to the prevention of blindness in developing countries seeking to eliminate the causes of avoidable blindness: cataract, trachoma, onchocerciasis, and childhood blindness; reduce the cost of eye care in developing countries; and create a network of highly efficient, productive, and self-sustaining eye hospitals that treat all persons, including the poorest.

Activities and programs

SightReach® Prevention

IEF works in Africa with the National Onchocerciasis Programs in Malawi and Cameroon to eliminate the disease, bringing the drug Mectizan® to approximately 2 million people annually. The IEF's childhood blindness and vitamin-A deficiency control initiatives distribute vitamin-A capsules to thousands of children through its child survival programs. The IEF also assists clinics in improving their services for children through training specialists, improving pediatric eye surgery and refractive services.

SightReach® Management

IEF provides leadership to apply innovations in management systems necessary for a paradigm shift in how eye care is delivered in the developing world. The IEF pioneered its sustainability strategy to help eye hospitals become more productive and self-sustaining, focusing on cataract treatment and quality of services. Since 1999, a network of government, public, NGO, and private eye clinics in 10 countries have adopted the SightReach® Management approach, dramatically increasing the number of people served, lowering costs, and increasing revenue while providing all patients with the same level of care.

SightReach Surgical®

Ophthalmologists in developing countries experience difficulty in purchasing needed equipment, instruments, and medical supplies because of the high cost, as well as the difficulty in procurement and shipping. To address this need, IEF established SightReach Surgical®, a non-profit online technology store that partners with ophthalmic product manufacturers to provide high-quality, low-priced products to eye care providers in the developing world. Since its establishment, SightReach Surgical® has grown dramatically, serving customers in over 40 countries in Africa, Asia, the Middle East, Latin America, and Eastern Europe.

For more information and to view the online catalog, go to www.sightreachsurgical.com or link through www.iefusa.org.

Kilimanjaro Centre for Community Ophthalmology (KCCO)

The KCCO is dedicated to the elimination of avoidable blindness through programs, training, and research, focusing on the delivery of sustainable and replicable community ophthalmology services.

Activities and programs

Program development aims

- Develop model community and hospital-based programs to reduce blindness from cataract and other VISION 2020 priority diseases.
- Develop programs aimed at improving the ability of existing eye care facilities to become self-sustaining.
- Help eye care professionals to develop, implement, and monitor district-based VISION 2020 plans.

Training

- Train ophthalmologists, ophthalmology residents, nurses, public health workers, and eye care program managers in community ophthalmology including needs assessment, program planning, management, and evaluation.
- Facilitate collaboration (north–south and south–south) with universities in Africa, Canada, Europe, Asia, and the USA to provide first-class training for current and future eye care service providers.

Research

- Investigate cost-effective ways to improve the uptake of, quality of, and satisfaction with eye care services.
- Provide technical support and training to researchers to undertake practical ophthalmological research in Africa.

Administration

The KCCO is part of Tumaini University and is associated with the Department of Ophthalmology at the Kilimanjaro Christian Medical College (KCMC) in Moshi, Tanzania. For more information, reports, and courses offered, please visit www.KCCO.net.

Korat Institute of Public Health Ophthalmology

Introduction

The Korat Institute of Public Health Ophthalmology was established in 1984 by the Ministry of Public Health of Thailand. It is attached to Maharat Nakhon Ratchasima Regional Hospital, 280 km northeast of Bangkok. The Korat Institute serves as the headquarters for the national program for prevention of blindness and serves as a regional training center for Southeast Asia and the western Pacific WHO region.

Activities and programs

Primary eye care in Southeast Asia was introduced through teaching and training of eye health care personnel at the Korat Institute. Manpower development, eye health system research, and development of an eye health information database are key areas of interest and activity. The Institute also plays a key role in technical cooperation between developing countries in the region, especially among the nations of Indochina. In close collaboration with WHO Collaboration Center for Prevention of Blindness, faculty from Jutendo University in Tokyo, Japan, assist the Korat Institute in hosting inter-country workshops.

A course in training mid-level eye care personnel in blindness prevention and eye care services is taught regularly at the Institute. This course has been taught in collaboration with Ramathibodi Faculty of Nursing, Mahidol University, and trains nurse practitioners in eye care for Thailand. It has now been upgraded to a regional course, inviting students from Indochina and Myanmar.

The Korat Institute is recognized for its regional eye care management course for ophthalmologists, which began in 1990. Taught every two years, it offers an intensive curriculum for both eye and public health professionals for training in management of blindness prevention and eye care system development.

Other activities include small incision cataract surgery training, low vision and refraction training, and training in pediatric ophthalmology.

The Korat Institute is a model center for technical cooperation in developing countries in eye care, personnel training, and training in management systems for Southeast Asia and the WHO western Pacific region.

Lions Clubs International Foundation

Introduction
Ever since Helen Keller challenged them to become Knights of the Blind in 1925, Lions have taken a special interest in the welfare of the blind and blindness prevention. Lions Clubs International Foundation (LCIF), the grant-making arm of Lions Clubs International, is especially committed to improving vision. Many LCIF grants help the visually impaired or deal with blindness prevention.

Activities and programs
Begun in 1989, LCIF's SightFirst program is the Lions' main blindness prevention initiative. SightFirst projects typically focus on strengthening eye care infrastructures and eye health delivery systems, training eye care workers, and intervening against the major blinding diseases through large-scale treatment initiatives.

SightFirst assists in restoring sight to the cataract blind, provides support for onchocerciasis programmes, and supports capital construction and renovation of eye clinics and hospitals, and works with local national organizations to provide training for eye health care workers. SightFirst works in collaboration with WHO to expand the effort to reduce the prevalence and incidence of blindness in children.

Campaign SightFirst II was launched in 2005 and will enable Lions to continue and expand the work of SightFirst. The goal is to raise at least US$150 million over a three-year period to combat preventable blindness.

For more information see:
www.lionsclubs.org (Lions Clubs International)
www.lcif.org (Lions Clubs International Foundation)

LV Prasad Eye Institute (LVPEI)

Aims and provisions
LV Prasad Eye Institute (LVPEI), Hyderabad, India, is a center of excellence in eye care services, basic and clinical research into vision-threatening conditions, and modes of management, training, product development, and rehabilitation for those with incurable visual disability. The main focus of all areas of work at LVPEI is to extend equitable and efficient eye care to all in need of care, especially disadvantaged populations in the developing world.

Established in 1987 and run by two non-profit trusts, LVPEI has come a long way in its journey toward realizing these goals. The LVPEI is a World Health Organization Collaborating Center in the area of blindness prevention, and houses the International Agency for the Prevention of Blindness (IAPB) Central Office.

Activities and programs
The Institute's activities are organized under six distinct arms: patient care services; research; training; community eye health; vision rehabilitation; and product development.

Patient care
The LVPEI offers services in all the subspecialties of the eye, including cornea, anterior segment, vitreous, retina, glaucoma, inflammatory eye diseases, and neuro-ophthalmology. Through all this, there is a focus on serving the needs of special groups, such as those with chronic diseases (e.g., diabetes), elderly patients, and children. The children's eye care center is staffed by professionals who understand the ramifications of eye disease and its management in newborns, infants, and growing children. Patients

whose visual disability cannot be cured are trained in the use of low-cost optical and non-optical aids to make best use of the vision they do have, at our Low Vision Center. Patients with total blindness are helped to achieve functional independence in our Rehabilitation Centers.

The Ramayamma International Eye Bank has had tremendous success in procuring and making corneas available for transplantation, both to corneal surgeons at LVPEI as well as several eye banks and surgical centers around India and elsewhere.

Training

Trained human resources represent a major need in developing countries. The LVPEI has become a world-renowned education center for all categories of eye care personnel from all over the world, who in turn are taking excellent eye care to many thousands of people in their countries. Education programs at LVPEI span short and long-term fellowships in all the ophthalmic subspecialties as well as optometry, nursing, equipment mainte-nance, vision techniques, and eye care management.

Research and product development

The LVPEI's robust research program has had many successes: research into stem cells and their transplantation to cure otherwise unmanageable eye diseases and conditions, and frontline research into the molecular genetic basis of eye diseases. On a very practical level, work at LVPEI has led to the development and routine production of large quantities of McKarey Kaufman corneal preservation medium, which is made available to eye banks and corneal transplantation centers across the sub-continent. Similarly, a variety of low-cost optical and non-optical devices have been made available for persons with low vision. On research, advocacy and training activi-ties, LVPEI collaborates with premier insti-tutions globally, ranging from the National Eye Institute and Lighthouse International in the USA to the International Centre for Eye Health in the UK and the University of New South Wales in Australia.

Community eye health

While the range of research and training activities is international, the focus is on bringing this quality of care to the poorest segments of India and the developing world. Successes include the establish-ment of rural eye health centers that provide high-quality eye care at the lowest possible cost – or at no cost – to those to whom such care would otherwise be inac-cessible. In fact, it is this same model that operates successfully in our nodal center in Hyderabad, Andhra Pradesh. At the LVPEI nearly 50% of our patients are treated free of cost.

Over the next few years, the LVPEI will progress toward its goal of building a sus-tainable network of eye care service delivery centers in the state of Andhra Pradesh as well as abroad. Efforts in this regard are already under way. The LVPEI has been instrumental in facilitating the development of both tertiary-care centers and secondary-care centers in India, and is also working with institutes in other devel-oping countries to develop infrastructure and human resources for sustainable eye care. Training, therefore, will continue to be a major area of focus, as will the emphasis on traditionally neglected areas such as rehabilitation and low vision care. The underlying philosophy of all these activities is equity, excellence, and efficien-cy in all aspects of eye care.

Nadi Al Bassar

Introduction

Nadi Al Bassar, Tunisia, was conceived in 1981, following the 7th Afro-Asian Congress of Ophthalmology, which was held in Tunis. Professor Ridha Mabrouk was the founder, together with a group of young volunteer ophthalmologists. It began as a small Center for Ophthalmology and Visual Science mainly for residents and ophthalmology students. Prevention of blindness soon became the main objective.

The discovery, in 1982, that 33% of the pupils at the School of the Blind were partially sighted led to the foundation of the low vision clinic, which offers free consultations. Nadi Al Bassar developed rapidly as a national non-governmental organization dedicated to the prevention of blindness and restoration of sight, one of the first to be thus established in a developing nation.

Activities and programs

Nadi Al Bassar awards scholarships to qualified students from Europe and the USA to study ophthalmic sciences. The Annual Al Bassar Course, in collaboration with the Faculty of Medicine, University of Tunis, attracts eminent speakers from American, European, and Japanese universities. As the center has grown and developed, ophthalmologists from the five Maghrebian countries (Libya, Algeria, Morocco, Mauritania, and Tunisia) have become active and involved. Tunisian ophthalmologists were awarded fellowships and advanced degrees from universities in the USA and Japan through Nadi Al Bassar.

Nadi Al Bassar has expanded its programs to include teaching and sharing therapeutic knowledge with its colleagues in neighboring countries including Mauritania, Libya, Sudan, and Iraq.

There has also been collaboration with other African countries. Similar projects were offered to South Africa and sub-Saharan West African countries including Senegal, Mali, Chad, Niger, Guinea, as well as Djibouti (on the Horn of Africa). The Faculty of Medicine, University of Tunis, signed twinning programs with some of these countries to receive ophthalmologists and residents for subspecialty training in Tunisia.

With experience and growth, Nadi Al Bassar developed into a donor NGO, joined the Partnership Committee of NGOs, became a full member of the International Agency of Prevention of Blindness, and was among the early supporters of VISION 2020.

Nadi Al Bassar now co-chairs EMR-North African Sub-Region, is active in the International Society of Geographical Ophthalmology, and is a member of the Foundation of the American Academy of Ophthalmology Committee.

Nadi Al Bassar can play an important role in prevention of blindness and restoration of sight in North Africa by continuing its work in advocacy, teaching, and regional outreach.

ORBIS International

Introduction

ORBIS International celebrated its 25th anniversary on 1 March 2007. Beginning in 1982 with a DC-8 aircraft converted to a flying eye hospital, ORBIS embarked on a program to teach appropriate surgical skills to eye doctors across the world. In many countries, ORBIS was responsible for the introduction of the operating micro-scope in eye surgery and introducing new techniques in cataract, retina, glaucoma, and pediatric eye disease. In 1994 ORBIS replaced the original Flying Eye Hospital with a wide-body DC-10 to continue this work. Also in the mid-1990s, ORBIS began establishing permanent in-country blindness prevention programs in Ethiopia, India, Bangladesh, China, and Vietnam. In 2003, recognizing the opportunity to maintain ongoing contact with doctors and partner institutions worldwide, ORBIS initiated Cyber-Sight, a telemedicine initiative which has created an extended ORBIS presence online for education and patient management. Working on a model of advocacy, capacity building, and sustainability, ORBIS strives to work with local partners to help them in their work towards the eradication of preventable blindness.

Mission

ORBIS is a non-aligned, non-profit global development organization whose mission is to preserve sight by strengthening the capacity of local partners in their efforts to prevent and treat blindness.

Activities and programs

The Flying Eye Hospital

The ORBIS Flying Eye Hospital (FEH) conducts 2- to 3-week programs in developing countries after being invited by the government and with the cooperation of local institutions and doctors acting as hosts. The permanent ORBIS FEH staff of 25, including doctors, nurses, technicians, and mechanics, is joined at each program by volunteer surgeons who donate their time to demonstrate surgery and to teach, both on the FEH and in local hospitals. The FEH classroom accommodates 50 host-country doctors who are able to view live surgery via a state-of-the-art audiovisual system, asking questions of the operating surgeons as the cases progress. A fully equipped examination/treatment room is available for a variety of activities, including laser treatment, and a recovery room is available to support patients before and after surgery.

Country Programs

Recognizing the need to emphasize capacity building and program sustainability, ORBIS has established long-term country programs in five countries. The first of these programs was in Ethiopia, where blindness from trachoma is endemic. Through the efforts of ORBIS, the WHO SAFE (**S**urgery, **A**ntibiotics, **F**acial cleanliness and **E**nvironmental improvements) strategy is being implemented to work toward the eradication of trachoma in that country. The strategy has been a model for other countries facing this terrible disease. Further ORBIS programs have been effective elsewhere, for example in India, where centers for pediatric eye care are being set up; in Vietnam, for the diagnosis and treatment of retinopathy of prematurity; and in Central America, where, with the cooperation of St. Jude Children's Research Hospital and the University of Tennessee, ORBIS has established a center of excellence for the diagnosis and treatment of childhood eye cancer (retinoblastoma).

Cyber-Sight®

The explosion in information technology in the 21st century has provided ORBIS with both an opportunity and a challenge. Recognizing the opportunity and accepting the challenge, ORBIS has established Cyber-Sight® as a means of maintaining close contact with partners established through traditional FEH programs and through in-country activities. Using the power of the Internet, through Cyber-Sight® ORBIS is now providing educational resources and support with patient consultation on a daily basis to partners heretofore limited to contact only when a formal ORBIS activity was physically present.

Organization

ORBIS is a dynamic organization with program offices in Addis Ababa, New Delhi, Dhaka, Shanghai, and Hanoi, and administrative offices in New York, London, Ottawa, Taipei, and Hong Kong. ORBIS activities take place in all parts of the developing world where blindness is a scourge.

The ORBIS Flying Eye Hospital is flown by volunteer pilots and maintained by both staff and volunteer mechanics. ORBIS is an integrated team of diverse individuals with complementary talents, all working towards the single goal of eliminating unnecessary blindness.

Francis I Proctor Foundation for Research in Ophthalmology

Introduction

The Proctor Foundation is an organized research unit at the University of California, San Francisco (UCSF). It has been closely associated with the Department of Ophthalmology since its establishment in 1947 to support eye research to find a cure for trachoma. Since then, the Foundation has evolved into one of the preeminent teaching and research facilities in the United States in the areas of infectious and inflammatory diseases of the eye. Even though the Foundation is an integral part of the University of California, it receives no state funds and is supported primarily by grants from the National Institutes of Health (NIH) and other extramural sources, by private donations, and by income from the original Proctor bequest.

Mission

This unique position of the Foundation within the University of California has allowed the Proctor Foundation to become one of the few institutions in the world with a significant commitment to blindness research in developing countries. Ninety percent of blind and visually disabled individuals are in developing countries where health care resources and research facilities are most limited. This is a primary area of the Foundation's research activity. The overall mission of the Proctor Foundation is threefold: education; patient care; and research.

Activities and programs
Education
The Proctor Foundation conducts a fellowship training program in cornea, external diseases of the eye, and uveitis. It accepts three North American fellows a year into

the program and a fourth specializing in uveitis. All fellows receive an intense program of surgical training as well with various members of the faculty. One or two foreign fellows are also accepted each year with the support of the Cecelia Vaughan Endowment. These fellows are observers only. All fellows in the program are required to complete a two-month course in epidemiology and clinical trials conducted by the Department of Epidemiology and Biostatistics at UCSF. They are also expected to complete and publish research projects during their fellowship training and to participate in all the weekly conferences and attend all the lectures throughout the year. The staff of the Proctor Foundation also trains UCSF ophthalmology residents and medical students as well as mentoring medical students from UCSF and other universities who apply to participate in our international research projects in the field in Ethiopia and India.

Research
The research activities of the Proctor Foundation consist of both laboratory-based research at UCSF and epidemiological research and clinical trials in the field in developing countries. The Proctor Foundation has a Clinical Microbiology Laboratory, the Heintz Virology Laboratory, the Kimura Ocular Immunology Laboratory, and the Chlamydial Research Laboratory. The Proctor International Center is presently conducting a large clinical trial which is monitoring the treatment of trachoma in Ethiopia. It is also conducting a prospective placebo-controlled clinical trial in Madurai, India, to test the efficacy of topical steroids in improving the visual outcome of patients with bacterial corneal ulcers.

Seva Foundation

Mission
Seva Foundation was founded in 1978 by a group of former World Health Organization smallpox campaign workers and their friends. They came together to prevent and relieve suffering through compassionate and effective action.

Activities and programs
The Sight Programs are the most enduring of Seva's activities. They are developed and funded jointly by Seva Foundation and Seva Canada Society. To achieve Sight Program goals, Seva does the following:

- Uses a public health approach to provide the best care for the most people, in which no one is turned away from services if they cannot pay.
- Provides training for local people in clinical skills and program management.
- Provides programs with start-up funding and equipment.
- Links professional volunteers as mentors to their program counterparts.
- Helps programs produce their own equipment and supplies to lower the cost of care.
- Helps partners work toward self-sufficiency.

Seva and partners establish systems to provide high-quality services to a large number of people. The methods used are sustainable to the maximum extent possible. Seva is a leader in developing strategies for sustainability in leadership, management, clinical services, materials, and funding. An active volunteer and exchange program ensures that experts from around the world get to learn from one another to improve service quality.

Nepal

For the past 27 years, Seva has worked with Nepal's Society for Comprehensive Eye Care, the WHO, and a team of national and international NGOs to develop a network of eye care services. This program is based upon results from the ground-breaking 1981 national blindness survey organized by Seva. Seva partners have been among innovators of safe extra-capsular cataract extraction with intraocu-lar lens implant in rural settings. Annual training workshops conducted by Nepali and Seva volunteer ophthalmologists and managers help disseminate surgical and community organizing strategies to centers throughout the country.

India

Over the years, Seva has assisted its principal partner in India, the Aravind Eye Care System, with research on barriers to surgery, subsidies for patient food and transport, construction, equipment donations, and technical consultation. Seva has partnered with Aravind to establish the Lions Aravind Institute for Community Ophthalmology (LAICO) to train eye workers from around the world. In recent years, Seva has worked with Aurolab and partner organizations to develop local production of intraocular lenses that enable cataract patients around the world to have near-perfect vision with the lens implant. Later, a multi-organiza-tion support team aided Aurolab's develop-ment of suture manufacture to make this vital supply available at a price most devel-oping country programs could afford. Along with Aravind, Seva has reached into other underserved regions of Asia to provide training of surgeons, ophthalmic assistants, field program coordinators, and managers, and has sponsored community-based eye services. Aravind often provides training and consultation to strengthen Seva partners.

Sadguru Netra Chikitsalaya, Chitrakoot

Seva has linked with this rural eye hospital to successfully expand the volume of cataract services, increase sustainability, and develop community-based programs.

Tibet

During the past 10 years Seva has worked with the public health bureau and staff of several eye hospitals in Tibet to improve the quality and volume of cataract surgery. Partner training has taken place in Nepal, at the Lumbini Eye Hospital, and during surgical eye camps in Tibet. The goal is to strengthen the network of eye services, beginning with cataract. In addition to providing training, equipment, and supplies for selected eye departments, Seva coordinated the first multi-prefecture assessment of the causes and distribution of blindness in Tibet. These data are the basis for large-scale planning and service efforts for which the health bureau relies heavily on Seva guidance and expertise.

Cambodia

Seva has expanded its partnerships into the northwestern provinces of Siem Reap, Battambang, and Bantey Manchey, all in Cambodia. The objective is to develop a sustainable eye care program within the national health plan in collaboration with provincial hospitals and the Ministry of Health. Seva provides technical and surgical support through teams of trainers and consultants from partner hospitals in Nepal and India, to achieve high-volume, high-quality cataract surgeries. Seva sponsors training for eye doctors and nurses and has established training programs in Cambodia. In addition to developing rural eye centers, Seva sponsors surgical eye camps and com-munity screening programs.

Tanzania

Beginning in 2001 the Kilimanjaro Centre for Community Ophthalmology (KCCO), in Moshi, Tanzania, invited Seva to be among its four charter founding organizations. This program is expanding training for public health personnel needed to fight blindness. Its relationship with the major ophthalmology training programs in Africa positions the KCCO to rapidly increase effectiveness of Africa's scarce resources for eye care and blindness prevention. Seva sponsors training programs as well as community initiatives to increase services to women and children, and to enhance every patient's quality of care.

Center for Innovation in Eye Care

During 2005 Seva initiated this center to accelerate the development and promotion of effective eye care strategies in reaching rural communities, women, and children. The center focuses on filling in information and strategic gaps required for achieving the goals of the WHO and the IAPB initiative VISION 2020: The Right to Sight.

Sight Savers International

Since 1950, Sight Savers International (SSI), previously known as the Royal Commonwealth Society for the Blind, has been working with local partners to combat blindness in developing countries. During this time SSI has helped restore sight to more than 5 million people and has treated over 70 million for potentially blinding conditions. Sight Savers International also supports programs for the education and rehabilitation of those who are irreversibly blind.

Sight Savers International is a founding member of VISION 2020: The Right to Sight, an international partnership of eye care agencies and the World Health Organization, which aims to eliminate

avoidable blindness by the year 2020 and to prevent 100 million people from going blind. The vast majority of blind people live in developing countries. Sight Savers International works with local partners in 30 of the poorest countries in the world to ensure that services are developed that are appropriate to local needs.

Activities and programs

Eye care

The programs supported by SSI include the following:

- Disease control, especially cataract surgery but also many other activities such as primary eye care, onchocerciasis, and trachoma control.
- Training of ophthalmic personnel.
- Development of infrastructure including refurbishment of eye units and provision of appropriate equipment and consumables.

Social inclusion

Blind and low-vision people are often marginalized within their own communities, and are consequently among the very poorest and most disadvantaged. While prevention and cure of blindness is SSI's main focus, it also aims to promote the social inclusion of visually impaired people through the following means:

- Support to community-based rehabilitation and inclusive education programs.
- Advocacy for the rights of visually impaired people.
- Researching evidence of the economic, social, and poverty alleviation impact of the work we support.

Operational research and impact

Sight Savers International recently increased resources to operational research in order to enhance policy and program development and is introducing improved mechanisms for assessing the impact of the programs it supports. More information can be obtained from the website at www.sightsavers.org, which has current information about the work in South Asia, the Caribbean, as well as West, East, Central, and Southern Africa. Current partners include Bangladesh, Belize, Benin, Cameroon, Gambia, Ghana, Guinea (Conakry), Guyana, Haiti, India, Jamaica, Kenya, Liberia, Malawi, Mali, Nigeria, Pakistan, Senegal, Sierra Leone, South Africa, Sri Lanka, Tanzania, Togo, Uganda, Zambia, and Zimbabwe.

World Health Organization (WHO)

Introduction
The WHO is the specialized agency for health of the United Nations System, established on 7 April 1948. It is an intergovernmental organization and receives its mandate from the member states, of which currently there are 192 members. The governing body at the headquarters level is the World Health Assembly(WHA) and the Executive Board (EB) and there are six Regional Committees, one each in the six WHO Regions. The WHA determines the governance of the Organization within the framework of WHO's constitution with the mandate to approve the WHO program and the related budget for each biennium and to make decisions on major policy issues.

Mission
The objective of the Organization, as stated in the constitution, shall be the attainment by all peoples of the highest possible level of health.

The overall functions of the Organization are spelt out in Article 2 of the constitution (see: www.who.int).

Activities and programs
WHO's role in Prevention of Blindness
Since the inception in 1978 of a WHO program dedicated to Prevention of Blindness (PBL) in pursuance to a WHA resolution (WHA 28.54, 1975), WHO has supported member states, to varying extents, in national program development within the context of strengthening national health systems to deal with the priority local eye health needs. Eye health delivery is seen as an integral part of the national health system based on the principles and practice of primary health care. The concept and practice of primary eye care have been actively promoted.

The following general strategies and tasks are carried out to further the objectives stated above:

- Articulating consistent, ethical and evidence-based *policy* and *advocacy* positions.
- *Managing information* by assessing trends and comparing performance; setting the agenda for, and stimulating, research and development.
- Catalyzing change through *technical and policy support*, in ways that stimulate cooperation and action and help build sustainable national and intercountry capacity.
- Negotiating and sustaining national and global *partnerships*.
- Setting, validating, monitoring and pursuing the proper implementation of *norms* and *standards*.
- Stimulating the development and testing of new *technologies*, *tools* and *guidelines* for disease control, risk reduction, health care management, and service delivery.

Global Elimination of Trachoma (GET 2020)

WHO constituted the WHO Alliance GET 2020 to provide a forum for collaboration and science-based technical support to member states in their goal to eliminate blinding trachoma. Promoting the use of the SAFE strategy (**S**urgery, **A**ntibiotics, **F**acial cleanliness and **E**nvironmental improvement), the Alliance meeting provides a forum for exchange of programmatic and research information among member states, NGOs, academic institutions etc. as well as for setting goals indicators and monitoring progress.

WHO's role in onchocerciasis control

Three major WHO programs summarize the international community's response towards onchocerciasis.

- Onchocerciasis Control Programme (OCP).
- African Programme for Onchocerciasis Control (APOC).
- Onchocerciasis Elimination Program for the Americas (OEPA).

WHO in VISION 2020: the Right to Sight

WHO in partnership with IAPB launched the Global Initiative for the Elimination of Avoidable Blindness in 1999. WHO brings to this collaborative effort all its normative functions and strategies outlined above. The WHA resolution 56.26 (2003) and the establishment of a VISION 2020 monitoring committee is a case in point. WHO meets on a regular basis with the Board of Trustees of IAPB, works closely with member countries and facilitates the collective efforts of the member states, NGOs, academic bodies and other civil society organizations.

Non-governmental organizations in official relations with WHO

WHO also facilitates through the Civil Service Initiative, relations between WHO and non-governmental and civil society organizations. The objectives of WHO's relations with NGOs are to promote the policies, strategies and activities of WHO and, where appropriate, to collaborate with NGOs in jointly agreed activities to implement them. The NGO Group members for Onchocerciasis Control set up in 2003 is a good example. The Lions Clubs International Foundation-funded Global Project for Elimination of Childhood Blindness, with WHO as the implementing agency, is another example, among others of such collaboration.

WHO Collaborating Centers

By definition a WHO Collaborating center (WHO CC), so designated by WHO, forms part of an inter-institutional collaborative network which supports the program at the country, intercountry, regional, interregional and global levels as appropriate. A WHO CC also participates in the strengthening of country resources, in terms of information, services, research and training in support of national health development.

There are several WHO CC linked to prevention of blindness in the different WHO regions. Examples of direct collaborative projects between WHO and Collaborating centers include a joint program with the National Eye Institute, National Institutes of Health, Bethesda, MD, USA.

For more information see:
http://www.who.int/en/
http://www.who.int/pbd/en/

West Virginia University International Health Program (IHP)

Mission

The mission of the International Health Program (IHP) at West Virginia University (WVU) is to foster learning, collaboration, and service in the global health community. The IHP provides opportunities to WVU faculty and students in international health environments in order to expand their knowledge of health care delivery systems, public health programs, and medical education systems in developing countries. The IHP strives to expand collaborative interdisciplinary research and share experiences of the United States and countries abroad to promote health worldwide. While providing service to residents in developing countries, WVU participants in IHP-affiliated sites abroad also gain cultural awareness and a spirit of cooperation with other countries.

Activities and programs

There are formal student/faculty exchange agreements with institutions in Barbuda, China, Guatemala, Italy, Mexico, Peru, and Uganda, which enable medical and pharmacy students to visit clinics and hospitals in these countries.

The mission of the IHP also includes providing a fully accredited Clinical Tropical Medicine and Parasitology Course to health care professionals. The course is offered every summer to applicants throughout the United States and abroad. The Clinical Tropical Medicine and Parasitology Course is held at WVU each summer and is one of seven United States institutions accredited by the American Society of Tropical Medicine and Hygiene (ASTMH). This course began in 1996 and is offered to all health care professionals in the USA and beyond. Physicians and registered nurses who complete the course are then eligible to sit for a certifying exam conducted by the ASTMH. Those who pass the certifying exam receive a Certificate of Knowledge in Clinical Tropical Medicine and Travelers Health.

Appendix H
Address book

Aravind Eye Hospital and Centers
Lions Aravind Institute of Community
Ophthalmology
1, Anna Nagar
Madurai 625 020
Tamil Nadu
INDIA
fax: +91 452 530 984
email: aravind@aravind.org;
eyesite@avavind.org
fax: +91 (0) 452-253 0984
www.aravind.org

Aurolab
Aravind Eye Hospital
1, Anna Nager
Madurai, Tamil Nadu 625 020
INDIA
email: sales@aurolab.com
fax: +91 (452) 253 5274
www.aurolab.com

Edna McConnell Clark Foundation
250 Park Avenue
New York, New York 10177-0026
USA
tel: 1 212 551 9100

Dana Center for Preventive
  Ophthalmology
Wilmer 122
Johns Hopkins Hospital
600 North Wolfe Street
Baltimore, MD 21287
USA
tel: 1 800 215 6467

Department of Ophthalmology
University of Melbourne
Eye Health Promotion Unit
32 Gisborne Street
East Melbourne, Victoria 3002
AUSTRALIA
http://cera.unimelb.edu.au

Department of Preventive and Tropical
  Ophthalmology
University of Munich
(Ludwig-Maximilians Universitaet
  Munchen)
Mathildenstrasse 8
80336 Munich
GERMANY
email: augenklinik@
med.uni-muenchen.de
fax: +49 89 5160 4942

Federation Internationale des
  Associations Catholiques d'Aveugles
2 Impasse de la Place
91100 Corbeil-Essonnes,
FRANCE
fax +33 1 60 89 49 46
email: fidaca@aol.com

Foresight
C/O Save Sight Institute
Sydney Eye Hospital Campus
GOP Box 6337
Sydney
NSW 2001
AUSTRALIA
fax: +61 29 382 7318
email: foresight@eye.usyd.edu.au

Foundation of the American Academy of Ophthalmology
FAAO International Assistance
655 Beach Street
San Francisco, CA 94109-1336
USA
email: wovaitt@aao.org
www.faao.org

Foundation Dark and Light
P.O. Box 672
3900 AR Veenendaal
NETHERLANDS
fax: +31 318 561 577
email: info@darkandlight.org
www.darkandlight.org

The Fred Hollows Foundation (FHF)
Locked Bag 3100
Burwood NSW 1805
AUSTRALIA
fax: +61 2 8338 2100
email: fhf@hollows.org
www.hollows.org

Fundación Oftalmológica Argentina Jorge Malbran
Azcuénaga 1077 2B,
1115, Buenos Aires,
ARGENTINA
tel: 54 1 814 4845
fax: 54 1 814 4853
email: ocroxatto@elsitio.net

Health for Humanity
415 Linden Avenue, Suite B
Wilmette, Illinois 60091
USA
fax +1 847 425 7901
email: information@healthfor
humanity.org
www.healthforhumanity.org

Healthlink Worldwide
Cityside
40 Adler Street
London E1 1EE
UK
fax: +44 20 7539 1580
email: info@healthlink.org.uk
www.healthlink.org.uk

Helen Keller International (HKI)
352 Park Avenue South, 12th Floor
New York, New York 10010
USA
fax: +1 212 532 6014
www.hki.org

HelpAge International
PO Box 32832
London N1 9ZN
UK
tel: +44 20 7278 7778
fax: +44 20 7713 7993
email: hai@helpage.org
www.helpage.org

InFOCUS
327 Tealwood Drive
Houston, Texas 77024
USA
fax: +1 713 468 7704
email: info@infocusonline.org
www.infocusonline.org

Institut d'Ophtalmologie Tropicale Africaine
Bamako
MALI
email: iota@iotaoccge.org
www.iotaoccge.org

International Agency for the Prevention of Blindness (IAPB)
IAPB Secretariat
LV Prasad Eye Institute
KV. Prasad Marg
Banjara Hills
Hyderabad 500 034
INDIA
fax: +91 40 354 8271
email: IAPB@lvpei.org
www.iapb.org

International Centre for Eye Health (ICEH)
London School of Hygiene and Tropical Medicine
Keppel Street
London WC1E 7HT
UK
www.jceh.co.uk
www.iceh.org.uk

International Council for Education of People with Visual Impairment (ICEVI)
Nandini Rawal Blind People's Association
Dr. Vikram Sarabhai Road
Vastrapur
Ahmedabad 380 015
INDIA
fax: +91 79 630 0106
email: larry@obs.org
www.icevi.org

International Eye Foundation (IEF)
10801 Connecticut Avenue
Kensington, Maryland 20895
USA
email: info@iefusa.org
fax: 240 290 0269
www.iefusa.org

International Organization Against Trachoma
Clinique Ophtalmologique Universitaire
Hôpital Intercommunal
40 Avenue de Verdun 9400
Creteil
FRANCE

International Orthoptic Association
Josephsplatz 20
D-90403 Nurnberg
GERMANY
fax: + 49 911 205 9612
www.internationalorthoptics.org

International Trachoma Initiative (ITI)
441 Lexington Avenue, Suite 1600
New York, New York 10017
USA
fax: +1212 490 6461
www.trachoma.org

Joint Commission on Allied Health Personnel In Ophthalmology
(JCAHPO)
2025 Woodlane Drive
St. Paul, Minnesota 55125-2995
USA
fax: +1 612 731 0410
email: Jcahpo@jcahpo.org

Kilimanjaro Centre for Community Ophthalmology (KCCO)
Tumaini University
P.O. Box 2254
Moshi
Tanzania
fax: +255 27 275 4890
email: kcco@kcco.net

Lighthouse International
111 East 59th Street
New York, New York 10022
USA
tel: +1 212 821 9705
email: info@lighthouse.org

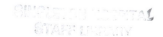

Lions Aravind Institute of Community Ophthalmology (LAICO)
72, Kuruvikaran Salai
Gandhinagar
Madurai, Tamil Nadu 625 020
INDIA
email: thulsi@aravind.org
fax: +91 (452)253 0984
www.aravind.org

MAP International
2200 Glynco Parkway
Brunswick, Georgia 31525-6800
USA
tel: +1 800 225 6800
www.map.org

Mekong Eye Doctors (MED)
Biesbosch 217
118JL
Amstelveen
NETHERLANDS
tel: +020 647 3879
info@mekongeyedoctors.nl

Micronutrient Forum
ILSI Human Nutrition Institute
One Thomas Circle NW
Washington, DC 20005-5802
USA
tel: +1 202 659 9024
fax: +1 202 659 3617
mnforum@Ilsi.org
www.micronutrientforum.org

Nadi al Bassar
9 Boulevard Bab Menara
1008 Tunis
TUNISIA
tel: +216 71 561 737
email: Nadi.albassar@planet.tn

National Eye Institute (NEI)
National Institutes of Health
31 Center Drive MSC 2510
Bethesda, Maryland 20892
USA
email: 2020@nei.nih.gov
www.nei.nih.gov

Norwegian Association of the Blind and Partially Sighted (NABP)
PB 5900
Hedgehaugen 0306
Oslo 3
NORWAY
fax: + 47 22 607 054
email: info@blindeforbundet.no

Oeil sur les Tropiques/ Oog vor de Tropen (OST)
Italielei 98
B2000 Antwerp
BELGIUM

Operation Eyesight Universal (OEU)
4 Parkdale Crescent NW
Calgary, Alberta TSN 3T8
CANADA
fax: +1-403-270-1899
www.giftofsight.com

ORBIS International, Inc.
520 Eighth Avenue, 11th floor
New York, New York 10018
USA
fax: +1-646-6745599
email: executive@ny.orbis.org
www.orbis.org

Organisation pour la Prevention de la Cécité (OPC)
17 Villa Alesia,
75014 Paris,
FRANCE
fax: +33 1 40 61 01 99
email: opc@opc.asso.fr

Organización Nacional de Ciegos de
   España (ONCE)
Ortega y Gasset 18
28006 Madrid
SPAIN
fax: +34 1 575 6053
email: efd@once.es

Overbrook School for the Blind
6333 Malvern Avenue
Philadelphia, Pennsylvania 19151-2597
USA
tel: +1-215-877-0313
email: bmk@obs.org
www.obs.org

Perkins School for the Blind
175 Beacon Street
Watertown, Massachusetts 02172
USA
tel: +1-617-924-3434
fax: +1-617-926-2027
www.perkins.org

Francis I Proctor Foundation for
   Research in Ophthalmology
University of California, San Francisco
95 Kirkham
San Francisco, CA 94143-0944
USA
www.ucsf.edu/proctor

Royal National Institute for the Blind
   (RNIB)
105 Judd Street
London WC1H 9NE
UK
fax: +44-20 7388 2034
email: helpline@rnib.org.uk
www.rnib.org.uk

Seva Foundation
1786 Fifth Street
Berkeley, CA 94710
USA
fax: +1-510-845-7410
email: sgilbert@seva.org
www.seva.org

Sight and Life
P.O. Box 2116
4002 Basel
SWITZERLAND
fax: +41 61 688 1910
email: sight.life@dsm.com
www.sightandlife.org

Sightfirst
Lions Clubs International
300 22nd Street
Oak Brook, Illinois 60521-8842
USA
email: lcif@lionsclubs.org
www.lionsclubs.org

Sight Savers International (SSI)
Grosvenor Hall
Bolnore Road
Haywards Heath
West Sussex RH16 4BX
UK
fax: +44-1444 415 866
email: generalinformation@sightsavers.org
www.sightsavers.org.uk

Society for Blindness Prevention
   Overseas (ZIEN/SBO)
P.O. Box 555
Spruitenbosstraat 6
2012 LK Haarlem
THE NETHERLANDS
fax: +31 23 532 8538

Surgical Eye Expeditions International,
   Inc. (SEE)
27 East De la Guerra Street, 2C
Santa Barbara, CA 93101
USA
fax: +1-805-965-3564
email: seeintl@seeintl.org
www.seeintl.org

Swedish Association of the Visually
  Impaired
(Synskadades Riksforbund)
Sandsborgsvagen 52
122 33 Enskede
SWEDEN
email: webbredaktor@srfriks.org
www.srfriks.org

Swedish Organization of Handicapped
  International Aid Foundation (SHIA)
P.O. Box 4060
102 61 Stockholm
SWEDEN
www.shia.se

Teaching Aids at Low Cost (TALC)
P.O. Box 49
St. Albans
Hertfordshire, AL1 5TX
UK
fax: +44-1727 846 852
email: talc@talcuk.org
www.talc@talcuk.org

Unite for Sight, Inc.
31 Brookwood Drive
Newtown, CT 06470-1842
USA
www.uniteforsight.org

Vision Aid Overseas (VAO)
12 The Bell Centre
Newton Road
Manor Royal
Crawley, RH10 2 FZ
UK
fax: +44-1293 535 026
www.vao.org.uk

Volunteer Eye Surgeons International
  Ltd, (VESI)
375 East Main Street
Bay Shore, NY 11706
USA
www.vesi.org

World Blind Union (WBU)
Canadian National Institute for the Blind
(CNIB)
1929 Bayview Avenue
Toronto, Ontario M4G 3E8
CANADA
www.worldblindunion.org

World Health Organization (WHO)
Program for the Prevention of
Blindness and Deafness
Headquarters
Avenue Appia
1211 Geneva 27
SWITZERLAND
tel: +41 22791 21 11
fax: +41 22 791 47 72
email: whopbd@who.int
www.who.int

Africa Regional Office
Parirenyatwa Hospital
P.O. Box BE 773
Harare
ZIMBABWE
tel: +263 4 07 69 51 / 4 70 74 93
fax: +263 4 79 01 46 / 4 79 12 14

Americas Regional Office
Pan American Sanitary Bureau
525 23rd Street NW
Washington, DC 20037
USA
tel: +1-202-8613200
fax: +1-202-2235971

Eastern Mediterranean Regional Office
P.O. Box 1517
Alexandria 21511
EGYPT
tel: +20 3 482 0223 / 482 0224 / 483 0090
fax: +20 3 483 8916

Europe Regional Office
8 Scherfigsvej
2100 Copenhagen
DENMARK
tel: +45 39 17 17 17
fax: +45 39 17 18 18

Southeast Asia Regional Office
World Health House
Indraprastha Estate
Mahatma Gandhi Road
New Delhi 110002
INDIA
tel: +91 11 331 7804 / 331 7823
fax: +91 11 331 8607 / 332 7972

Western Pacific Regional Office
PO Box 2932
Manila 1099
PHILIPPINES
tel: +63 2 528 8001
fax: +63 2 521 1036

Appendix I

References and Resources

This list of publications, manuals for training and management, and visual aids is of particular interest to people involved in sight restoration and blindness prevention in disadvantaged populations. The list is not exhaustive. Please use the address book to contact organizations involved in publication of these various materials.

Comprehensive

Gilbert C., Raman U., Francis V. (ed.) *World Blindness and its Prevention*. Vol 7. International Agency for the Prevention of Blindness, in collaboration with the World Health Organization, 2005.

Johnson G. J. *et al* (eds). *Epidemiology of Eye Disease*. 2nd ed. London: Edward Arnold; 2003.

Sandford-Smith J. *Eye Diseases in Hot Climates*. 4th ed. India: Elsevier, 2003

Sandford-Smith J. *Eye Surgery in Hot Climates*, 3rd ed. Leicester: F.A. Thorpe Publishing; 2004

Sutter E., Foster A., Francis V Hanyane. *A Village Struggles for Eye Health*. London: International Centre for Eye Health; reprinted 2002.

Tasman W. (ed). *Duane's Clinical Ophthalmology*. Chapters 50–67: Geographic and Preventive Ophthalmology. Philadelphia: Lippincott-Raven; updated annually.

Appropriate technology

Technology for VISION 2020. London: International Centre for Eye Health, 2005.

Technology Guidelines for a District Eye Care Programme. VISION 2020 Technology Working Group, 2006. Available through International Centre for Eye Health, London.

Standard List of Medicines, Equipment, Instruments, Optical Supplies, and Educational Resources. Updated every two years. International Centre for Eye Health, London.

Directory of Teaching and Information Resources for Blindness Prevention and Rehabilitation. 2nd ed. International Centre for Eye Health, London.

Epidemiology

Johnson G.J., Minassian D.C., Weale R. *The Epidemiology of Eye Disease*. 2nd ed. Arnold, 2003. Available (at discount price for developing countries only) from International Centre for Eye Health, London.

Causes and Magnitude of Blindness and Visual Impairment. World Health Organization, 2002. Available as download from the WHO website.

Primary eye care

Prevent Blindness Through Primary Eye Care. Geneva: International Eye Foundation and World Health Organization. Available as a download through WHO website.

Cataract

Cox I, Stevens S. *Ophthalmic Operating Theatre Practice: A Manual for Developing Countries.* London: International Centre for Eye Health, 2002.

Ruit S., Tabin G.C., Wykoff C.G. *Fighting Global Blindness: Improving World Vision through Cataract Elimination*. Washington D.C., American Public Health Association, 2006.

Rapid Assessment of Cataract Surgery Services and a Simplified Cataract Grading System. Available to download from the WHO website.

Leprosy

Courtright P., Johnson G. *Prevention of Blindness in Leprosy*. Geneva: Proctor Foundation, International Centre for Eye Health, and World Health Organization, 1988.

Courtright P., Lewallen S. *Guide to Ocular Leprosy for Health Workers: A Training Manual for Eye Care in Leprosy.* Singapore: World Scientific Publications, 1993.

Courtright P., Lewallen S. *Training Health Workers to Recognize, Treat, Refer, and Educate Patients about Ocular Leprosy.* Singapore: World Scientific Publications: 1993.

Low vision and rehabilitation

Keeffe J. *Assessment of Low Vision in Developing Countries. Book 2. The Effects of Low Vision and Assessment of Functional Vision.* Melbourne, Australia: University of Melbourne; 1994.

Werner D. *Disabled Village Children. A Guide for Community Health Workers, Rehabilitation Workers, and Families*. Palo Alto, California: The Hesperian Foundation, updated 2002.

Onchocerciasis

The Mectizan Program Notes. Published quarterly by The Mectizan Donation Program. View past editions and sign up to receive electronically at www.mectizan.org

WHO Expert Committee on Onchocerciasis. Technical Report Series no. 852. Geneva: World Health Organization, 1995.

WHO Criteria for Certification of Interruption of Transmission/ Elimination of Human Onchocerciasis. Geneva: World Health Organization, 2001. Document No: WHO/CDS/ CEE/2001.18a.

Trachoma

The following trachoma publications are available to download from the World Health Organization website:

Achieving Community Support for Trachoma Control.
Final Assessment of Trichiasis Surgeons.
Trachoma Control: A Guide for Programme Managers.
The SAFE Strategy.
Trichiasis Surgery for Trachoma.
Trachoma Epidemiological Survey Protocol.
Primary Health Care Management of Trachoma.
Guidelines for the Rapid Assessment of Blinding Trachoma.
Trachoma Grading Cards.

Vision 2020

Available at the World Health Organization website:

Vision 2020 CD. Developing an Action Plan to Prevent Blindness at National, Provincial and District Level.
Report of the First Five Years of Vision 2020.

Xerophthalmia and childhood blindness

Sommer A. *Vitamin A Deficiency and Its Consequences: A Field Guide to Detection and Control*. 3rd ed. Geneva: World Health Organization, 1995.

Sommer A, West K. *Vitamin A Deficiency: Health, Survival, and Vision*. New York: Oxford University Press, 1996.

Vitamin A Supplements: A Guide to Their Use in the Treatment and Prevention of Vitamin A Deficiency and Xerophthalmia. Geneva: World Health Organization, 1988.

Regular Publications

IAPB News. Hyderabad, India: International Agency for the Prevention of Blindness. [Free.]

Community Eye Health Journal. London: International Centre for Eye Health. [Subscription; free to readers from a developing country] English, French, Chinese.

River Blindness News. Atlanta, Georgia: The Carter Center. [Free.]

Sight and Life Newsletter incorporating the Xerophthalmia Club Bulletin *Sight and Life* Basel, Switzerland: DSM Nutritional Products [Free.]

Index

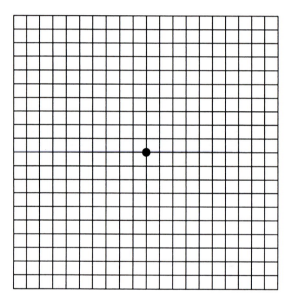

Amsler Grid for testing macular function. Each eye is tested separately. Cover the left eye first and direct the patient to look at the central dot at a distance of approximately 20 cm. Ask the patient what he/her sees around the dot while looking directly at the dot. Curved lines, distortion, and blank spaces are usually indicative of abnormal macular function. Repeat by testing left eye while covering right eye.